FoRePLaY

The Bedside Companion

FoRePLay

The Bedside Companion

Hugh de Beer, Al Kemp & Hilary Walton

HarperCollins*Publishers*

HarperCollins*Publishers*

25 Ryde Road, Pymble, Sydney, NSW 2073, Australia
31 View Road, Glenfield, Auckland 10, New Zealand

National Library of Australia
Cataloguing-in-Publication data:

De Beer, Hugh.
   Foreplay: the bedside companion.

   ISBN 0 7322 5078 1.

   1. Sex - Humor. 2. Sex - Miscellanea. I. Kemp, Al,
   1950- . II. Walton, Hilary. III. Title.

306.70207

Cover and internal illustrations by Sue Ninham
Cover design by Katie Ravich
Printed in Australia by McPhersons Printing Group,
Maryborough, Victoria

9 8 7 6 5 4 3 2 1
97 96 95 94

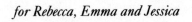

for Rebecca, Emma and Jessica

Preface

*Foreplay is the difference between making love
and having sex.*

A glass of champagne, a body massage, laughter, delicious anticipation ... What does foreplay mean to you?

Foreplay can be as exciting as sexual intercourse itself, and sometimes even more so. Foreplay equals sexy fun and games, and that's what you'll have if you follow our hints both in and out of your bedroom. All you need is a playmate, a sense of adventure and a wicked outlook.

Between these covers you will find an orgy of games, quizzes, trivia, recipes and fun to ignite your inventive spirit and spice up your love life. Immerse yourself in the erotic! Indulge yourself in our pages of suggestions, play the sexy games and try the teasing quizzes, concoct a dangerous lovers' cocktail or two ...

What turns you on? What are your partner's secret fantasies? Just how far would you go? *Foreplay: The Bedside Companion* will reveal fascinating facets of you and your partner. So delve between the covers and enjoy the steamy seductions offered in this book.

Contents

Aphrodisiacs

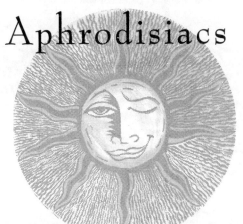

Powdered rhinoceros horn, deer sperm, dragon's blood, goat's testicles . . .

Sound appetising? Believe it or not, these weird and wonderful ingredients are famous as aphrodisiacs. (Of course, whether they actually work or not is another thing . . .)

An aphrodisiac is anything which incites sexual passion. If dragon's blood and goat's testicles sound like a little too much effort, simpler seductions like perfume, lacy underwear, and sexy films might just do the trick.

The word 'aphrodisiac' comes from Aphrodite, the Greek goddess of sexual love, who 'overcomes all mortal men and immortal gods with desire'. Aphrodite's first appearance was in the sea, where she was born in the foam, and floated ashore on a shell. Is it any wonder that the beach is the setting for many sexual encounters? Or that the French poet Valéry called swimming 'fornication with the wave'? The sight and smell of the sea, a place

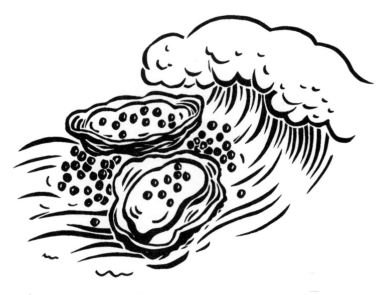

where we are usually more or less naked, is a powerful aphrodisiac.

Talk of the sea brings us to oysters, widely regarded as an aphrodisiac par excellence. Not only do oysters smell and taste of the sea, not only do they look slippery and plump and sexy, they also contain high amounts of trace elements and minerals, particularly zinc, iodine and phosphorus. Then there is caviar, or if your seduction budget is a small one, other fish eggs such as salmon 'caviar' or even the humble taramasalata. They all have that certain scent of the sea which is the prime ingredient in the aphrodisiac properties of these foods.

Many aphrodisiacs are extracted from plants and some of these are toxic, so be careful of narcotic and hallucinatory drugs with exaggerated reputations! Although they can produce a quick high, there are correspondingly rapid lows. Alcohol is a prime example—Shakespeare had his bawdy porter in Macbeth admit that alcohol 'provokes and unprovokes: it provokes the desire, but it takes away the performance.' A couple of drinks may increase excitement, sharpen intention and release the inhibitions, but there is a very fine line between the stimulation of a few drinks and the embarrassing inability to perform at all.

The seventeenth century herbalist Nicholas Culpeper suggested garlic, parsley and mint as sexual stimulants. Parsley has a high iron content, which should increase stamina; and both parsley and mint are good breath-sweeteners, a property not to be ignored when intent on seduction.

Truffles are notorious aphrodisiacs, probably because of the heavy musk component in their aroma. Musk is well-known as a 'carnal' scent. As with caviar, there are cheaper alternatives—try substituting some of the stronger flavoured wild mushrooms for truffles: cepes, chanterelles or dried shiitake for example.

In Asia, the durian fruit is considered a great aphrodisiac: 'When the durian falls, the sarongs rise.' For most Westerners, the rich custardy fruit is pleasant enough, but the overpoweringly faecal smell of the prickly skin is hardly a turn-on. Other fruits like the persimmon have semen-like overtones which appeal to some.

Chocolate is another well-known stimulant, and was said to be used by Montezuma, Casanova and Madame Du Barry to arouse their partners' desire. Our Chocolate lovers recipes provide delicious sweet treats for chocoholics throughout the book. Spices, by their very definition, are capable of hotting things up—chillies, curries, garlic and all manner of hot foods are valued throughout the world for their firepower. The hot element in chilli, capsaicin, burns the tongue's nerve endings, and a false pain message is sent to the brain. In response, the brain releases endorphins which act like a shot of morphine and create an exciting high. Our Hot Spots will give you plenty of spicy food ideas to keep your love life sizzling.

Some foods are suggestive because of their shape or appearance. In Italian, the slang for female genitals is the word for 'fig'. The avocado got its name from the Aztec for 'testicles'. Spear-like asparagus is suggestive, its effect heightened by the strong aroma. Mussels on the shell look like female genitals, while a ripe peach with its furry cleft looks like a bottom to some, or a symbol of female sex to others. As for bananas, not to mention carrots and cucumbers . . . Need we go on?

Find your own aphrodisiacs—you and your partner will have fun experimenting! Test out your favourite food and drinks on each other, tantalise with the touch of silk and velvet, wallow in your favourite film . . . A film or a book can do the trick. How about the combination of food and lechery in the film *Tom Jones*, where Albert Finney and Joyce Redman eat their food with explicit oral sex play. They never take their eyes off each other, and don't touch, but the effect is sizzling. Or there's the raw egg passed between the lovers' mouths in *Tampopo*, or the lust-making recipe of Quail with Rose Petals in *Like Water for Chocolate*.

There are no guarantees for a sure-fire aphrodisiac, but there is plenty of enjoyment in the search for one. Candlelight and champagne may trigger a response, but so can a picnic of pears and cheese. Experiment and explore, dabble in different paths to desire, and remember, the aphrodisiac, whatever it is, works if the ambience is right.

Here with a Loaf of Bread beneath the bough,
A Flask of Wine, a Book of Verse—and Thou
Beside me singing in the Wilderness
And Wilderness is Paradise enow.

Edward Fitzgerald, *Omar Khayyam*

★ ★

Chocolate lovers

Sweeten your love life with this seductive nightcap:

Hot Mocha Chocolate

1 tbsp instant coffee

1 tbsp cocoa

2 tsp coffee crystals (sugar)

2 cups hot water (boiling point)

whipped cream

chocolate curls

Combine coffee, cocoa and coffee crystals. Add boiling water and stir.
Pour into elegant serving cups and top with whipped cream
and chocolate curls.

★ ★

Between The Sheets

SEXY WORD CROSSWORD

This crossword is similar to Scrabble, where you have to build up words that fill a grid. All you need to play the game, however, is a die, a piece of paper and a pen or pencil. A good vocabulary of words with sexual meanings or connotations will also be helpful!

Simply draw your own grid on the paper. It can be any size, depending on how confident you are. If you want to add another dimension to the game, you might even make some of the squares 'rewards', so that a player putting a letter in that square, for instance, may be able to remove one of the other player's garments.

PLAYING THE GAME

Each player throws a die. The highest score goes first.
Words should have the same number of letters as shown on the die when it is thrown.
The players score a point for each letter they use in the grid. Each player has ten throws of the die. The highest score wins.

Our conscience obliges us to warn shy people of this aphrodisiac property of celery that they might abstain from eating it, or at least use it prudently. It is enough to stress that it is not in any way a salad for bachelors.

Giles MacDonogh, *Grimod de la Reyniere*

Asparagus . . . being taken fasting several mornings together, stirreth up bodily lust in man or woman, whatever some have written to the contrary.

Nicholas Culpeper, *Complete Herbal*

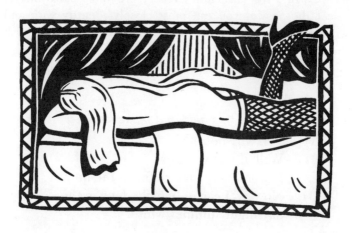

Those who wish to lead virtuous lives should abstain from truffles.

Old French Proverb

Buy a two-person split set of earphones for your Walkman, and listen to sensually rhythmic music as you lie in front of a wintertime log fire.

Pour a little massage oil into your lover's belly button. Use the tip of your finger to trace oily spirals on the stomach.

Keep a dream diary and write down your sexy dreams. Why not share them with your lover?

Use a vibrator to massage the whole body.

How Do You Rate As a Lover?

Do you turn your lover to jelly with your wild, untamed passion? Do you ooze sexuality? Or do you have the sexual prowess of a wet dishcloth? To explore your sexual image, select the answer you can most closely identify with and write it down on a piece of paper. When (or if . . .) you finish the quiz, go to the scores on page 168 to see how you rate.

1. Would you stop this quiz and make love now?
- A)   Yes, why not?
- B)   Well, if you want to . . .
- C)   It won't take long to finish the quiz.
- D)   No way, I can only make love in the day/night/summer/winter . . .

2. Describe how you would feel if someone told you that you weren't to make love for a year.
- A)   Where did I put that solo sex aid?
- B)   What's new?
- C)   Aaaagh!
- D)   Baffled, but I'd accept it.

3. Describe how you feel when you have an orgasm.
- A)   What's an orgasm?
- B)   Worried about the neighbours.
- C)   Like a cigarette.
- D)   The earth moves . . . and moves . . . and moves.

4. *Describe how your partner enjoys orgasm.*
   - A) I've never asked.
   - B) Who cares?
   - C) Deliriously, because they're with me.
   - D) Well, all that screaming must have meant something.

5. *Can your lover ask you to do things to them without fear or rejection?*
   - A) It depends what sorts of 'things'.
   - B) No—I'd be insulted if my lover asked me to do more.
   - C) I don't have to be asked, I know already.
   - D) Yes, anytime.

6. *What is the best part of your body?*
   - A) I haven't looked.
   - B) It depends on the day I'm having.
   - C) The whole package, of course!
   - D) The part I can't see in the mirror.

7. *What is your favourite sex manual?*
   - A) The instructions on a condom box.
   - B) *The Joy of Sex* or the *Kama Sutra*.
   - C) My own imagination.
   - D) The dictionary.

8. *If cars reflect the owner's sexuality, what sort of car would you be?*
- A)   A classy Jag or Rolls.
- B)   A red Ferrari or Porsche.
- C)   A Combi van.
- D)   A brown Datsun with fluffy dice.

9. *What do you think about directly after an orgasm?*
- A)   Who is going to sleep on the wet spot?
- B)   That was fantastic—I hope it was great for you too.
- C)   Did I put the cat out?
- D)   Let's do that again.

10. *What does foreplay mean to you?*
- A)   Kissing.
- B)   Checking to see that my partner is awake.
- C)   Playing with my partner's body for hours on end before we make love.
- D)   Is it something in chess?

11. *What is something erotic you'd do with a piece of fruit?*
- A)   Make fruit salad.
- B)   Rub the juice over parts of my lover's body and lick it off.
- C)   Dip pieces of it in hot melted chocolate and feed it to my lover.
- D)   Put it in the fridge and save it for breakfast.

12. *What one thing would you seek in a partner to make the perfect lover?*
    A) Compliments me all the time.
    B) A great imagination.
    C) Keeps socks on in bed.
    D) Is able to match my stamina.

13. *How do you feel if your partner gives you directions during lovemaking?*
    A) Great—I'm not a mindreader.
    B) There's only one boss.
    C) OK, but I thought I knew all the moves by now.
    D) Angry and insulted.

14. *What sort of 'afterplay' do you like?*
    A) Post mortem of the event: 'Was I OK?/Did you like it?'
    B) Sleeping.
    C) Just relaxing and talking together.
    D) Hugging and kissing.

15. *Do you vary your lovemaking positions?*
    A) On Christmas and birthdays.
    B) Never—why change something that works?
    C) Every time.
    D) Whenever the mood arises.

16. *What is your favourite surface to make love on?*
    A)   My partner's body.
    B)   Anywhere—we make it exciting
         wherever we are.
    C)   The back seat of a car.
    D)   A filing cabinet.

17. *Do you masturbate more than making love?*
    A)   Yes.
    B)   I don't masturbate—I might go blind.
    C)   No—my love life's enough of a handful.
    D)   No.

18. *Do you think it is important to help your lover reach
    an orgasm?*
    A)   My partner always reaches orgasm.
    B)   Yes, it's very important.
    C)   My partner is responsible for his/her own
         orgasm.
    D)   Why? Who cares as long as I enjoy
         myself?

19. *Does romance rate in your lovemaking?*
    A)   Yes, it's always there.
    B)   Get real—that stuff's only in books and
         films.
    C)   Yes of course—we're the greatest lovers
         of the 20th century.
    D)   As long as it doesn't take up too much
         time and effort.

20. How do others rate you as a lover?

    A)   Is 'as sexy as a brussel sprout' a
               compliment?
    B)   Great!
    C)   No one has complained yet.
    D)   Who cares?

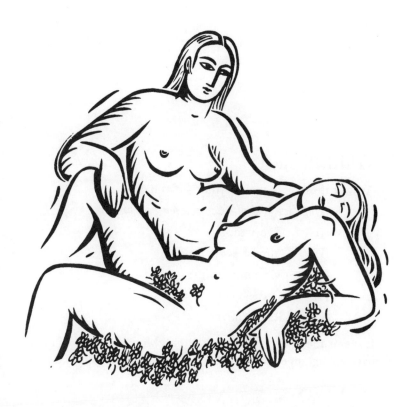

Truth or dare

Answer these with your partner—if you dare . . .

Do you ever fake an orgasm?

A)   Always

B)   Fairly often

C)   Occasionally

D)   Never

Most people fudge it at some time or another. 2% of both men and women agree that they always pretend to have orgasms. 41% of women (compared with 14% of men!) occasionally fake it, and 43% of women (compared with 81% of men) say they never fake.

Truth or dare

Answer these with your partner—if you dare . . .

When making love how often do you have an orgasm?

A)   Every time

B)   Almost every time

C)   Most of the time

D)   Occasionally

E)   Rarely/never

It seems the sexes really are different. More than 50% of men have an orgasm every time. Only 14% of women usually do.

❀ FAMOUS LOVERS ❀

*Dress up as your favourite pair of lovers through history,
and enjoy stripping away the layers . . .*

Antony and Cleopatra

Helen and Paris

Launcelot and Guinevere

Adam and Eve

Morticia and Gomez (*The Addams Family*)

Sleeping Beauty and Prince Charming

Scarlett O'Hara and Rhett Butler

Romeo and Juliet

Bonnie and Clyde

Rick and Ilsa (*Casablanca*)

*A quiz asking men what they most liked in bed revealed, to
nobody's surprise, that oral sex is top of the list. Here's the
ratings:*

1) Oral sex.

2) Vaginal squeezing.

3) Being teased just a little bit.

4) Hips that move: sex is about rhythm.

5) A bit of noise.

6) Participation: an active partner who will take the lead
   sometimes.

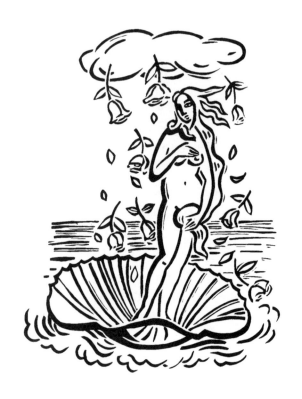

Madrigal

My love in her attire doth show her wit
It doth so well become her
For every season she hath dressings fit,
For Winter, Spring and Summer
No beauty she doth miss
When all her robes are on
But beauty's self she is
When all her robes are gone.

TRADITIONAL, COLLECTED 1602

The Rose

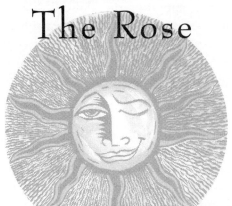

Roses have always been the flowers of love, as anyone who has sent or received a mass of long-stemmed red roses will tell you. It is not only the swoon-making scent of roses that make them such a popular expression of romantic love, but the way they bloom. Beginning with a small furled bud, roses slowly open into full-blown, spectacular beauty.

Not many flowers are attractive at all stages of flowering, but roses can be given as love-tokens as tiny pink buds, as partially opened blooms, or as the triumphant production of a fully flowered rose, its centre stamen fully visible.

Traditionally, roses have been used in medicines and food (rose hips are a source of vitamin C) as well as for fragrances. Rose oil is one of the most antiseptic of plant oils but it is the least toxic. Known in the fragrance industry as 'Attar of Roses', a legend tells us that it was discovered in the 1600s by Princess Nur Mahal, wife of the Emperor of Kashmir. Her servants would sprinkle rose petals in her bath, and one day she noticed a thin film of oil on the water. This was the pure essence of rose scent, and the princess had the oil collected and securely sealed into bottles.

Even in winter, when the rose is bare of blooms, the rose hips (the fruit left after the flowers disappear) of the different rose varieties can brighten the garden with a great range of colour. The rose's flowers are certainly beautiful and fragrant, but perhaps the ability of this plant to give year-round pleasure is also what couples it with love and romance in our imaginations.

The Book of Genesis never mentioned the rose as being in the Garden of Eden, but in one myth Eve was reputed to have kissed the white rose and made it blush with delight, transforming it into a pink rose. The Cappadocian father, Saint Basil 'The Great', said that the rose bush was without thorns right up to the time of the expulsion from the Garden of Eden. Other sources say that the rose bush was thornless until Adam devoured the forbidden apple, when they appeared to mark man's corruption.

The fascination for the rose in romance seems eternal. The Egyptian Queen, Cleopatra, was said to have greeted her triumphant Roman lover, Marc Antony, in a room filled with fifty centimetres of rose petals. There was no doubt that they were knee deep in love. And according to Shakespeare, Cleopatra soaked the sails of her ship in rose water when she sailed to meet Marc Antony.

The Roman Emperor Nero (37–68 AD) was so infatuated by the rose that he paid over four million sesterces (perhaps three hundred thousand dollars today) on roses to decorate one single banquet. Another fancy of Nero was the beautiful married woman Poppaea. He was so besotted by her loveliness that he vowed to see her naked in her bath. She managed to foil his lustful schemes, however, by floating vast amounts of rose petals on the surface of the water.

Perhaps the most famous of modern day love stories includes the sad and romantic icon Marilyn Monroe. After the death of the great movie star, her second husband, the legendary baseball star Joe DiMaggio, pledged to keep a black vase on her grave filled with fresh red roses twice a week—a measure of true love and devotion that would last forever.

The meaning of roses harks back to ancient legend, and is based on their colour. Red, as we know, means passion, love and faithfulness; white means purity and innocence, and is a symbol of peace; yellow roses usually represent true friendship. So give that special person a bunch of roses today with a secret floral message. Fill your boudoir with these exotic blooms, turn the lights down low and let them perfume your moments of passion together.

Roses feature in an old European test of a lover's faithfulness, in which a moss rose was picked on Midsummer's Eve, gently wrapped, and put away until Christmas Day, when it would be discreetly inspected. If the rose showed any signs of its original colour the lover was true, but if it had completely faded there would be no presents for Christmas.

A rose is a rose is a rogue

Tom Robbins

Between The Sheets

FINISH THE FANTASY

Roll the die and the highest score begins. Each number on the die is represented by one of the fantasies below.

Read out whatever number you get on the die and complete the fantasy.

1) *I had no choice but to lie back and enjoy the warmth of those hands caressing my body . . .*

2) *I've never been involved in a trio, and I wasn't going to let this opportunity pass . . .*

3) *Waiting outside my block of flats for a taxi, I couldn't help but notice through a bedroom window a couple making love . . .*

4) *I was going home on the train late at night. There was no one else on it, except for one gorgeous stranger who was looking straight at me . . .*

5) *There I was, stretched out naked on the bed, with my hands and feet tied. The door opened and my dominant partner entered, wearing . . .*

6) *The first time I made love was . . .*

Take a juicy mango, peach or orange and rub the juice all over your partner's belly. Then sensuously lick or wash the juice off.

Whisper sexy ideas into your lover's ear.

I
Who is your favourite singer?

II
Have you ever masturbated while talking to your lover on the telephone? Would you?

III
How would you rate oral sex as a form of foreplay?

Love Spells

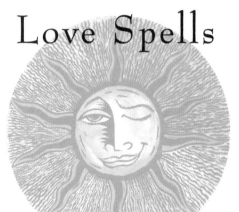

Can we make someone desire us by putting a spell on them? It might make our love lives a lot easier, and for centuries people believed that spells and charms did work. All we can say is, it won't hurt to try, and you never know . . .

Why not try some of these strange seductive spells? But remember, be careful what you wish for . . .

Cut an apple in half and place one half behind your bedroom door and the other half inside your clothes close to your heart. Think about the one you want all day, and if your desire is strong your lover will be standing at your bedroom door at midnight.

A piece of lemon peel is placed under the armpit for an evening. Think of the loved one as hard as you can. Next day, grind up the lemon peel and offer it to the one you want in some food or drink. They are guaranteed to fall madly in love with you.

Rub your bedpost with lemon peel and you will dream of your loved one.

Marigolds exert a powerful influence. Sow marigold seeds in a pot full of earth. The earth must have been walked on by the one that you care for. When the flowers grow, they are offered to the would-be love, who will be yours from then on.

Put a sprig of clover in your lover's shoe, and you will have a lover who is faithful even when travelling far away from you.

Marriages celebrated during a full moon will be full of happiness.

A couple of drops of your blood in someone's food or drink will make them fall in love with you.

Write down your name on a piece of paper, and the name of the one you want. Cross out all the letters your names have in common. Count the remainder of the letters while reciting 'Love, marriage, friendship, adoration.' See which one you end up on!

Count seven stars for seven nights. On the eighth day, the first person you shake hands with will be THE ONE.

A hazelnut with two kernels found on Hallowe'en: if the finder eats one kernel in silence and then manages to persuade an intended partner to eat the other, a long and faithful marriage will result.

Catch a snail and shut it in a box for the night. The silver trail it makes will show your lover's initial.

Gypsy girls wear an ivy leaf close to the heart when pursuing the love of their life. This is the chant they use:

Ivy, ivy, I love you,
In my bosom I put you,
The first young man who speaks to me
My future husband he shall be.

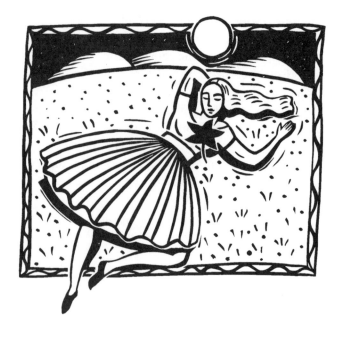

Take a lock of your lover's hair and place it in your right shoe, saying the following charm when the moon is new:

Bright moon, new moon,
Clear and fair,
Lift up my right foot,
See my love's hair.

Lift your right foot, think of your lover, and he or she will appear.

Summon your beloved by putting your shoes together at right angles, with the toe of one shoe touching the instep of the other. Say the charm:

When my true love I want to see
I shape my shoes into a T.

Tie one of your shoelaces into a knot and put it under your pillow while you say the charm:

This knot, this knot, this knot I tie,
To see my true love, this knot I tie
To see my love in his array
And what he walks in every day.
And if my love be dressed in green,
His love for me will always be seen
And if my love is dressed in blue
His love for me is ever true.

Sleep on the shoelace knot and see what happens in the morning.

Sit naked in front of a full-length mirror so that you can see yourself and a photograph of the one you desire. Do not look directly at the photograph but make sure you can see it in the mirror. Put on some scent or after-shave. Have seven pins, a candle and a red paper heart ready. Put one of the pins about half-way down the candle. Light the candle, and as it burns towards the pin gradually place the other six pins in the paper heart. Recite these words:

> *It is not this candle alone I stick*
> *But my lover's heart I mean to prick*
> *If (name) be asleep or (name) be awake,*
> *I'll have (name) come to me and speak.*

When the flame reaches the pin, take it out while it is still warm and stick it with the others in the red heart. By now the phone should be ringing with your intended lover on the line.

In Norfolk, a ladybird is known as a Barnaby, in local dialect pronounced 'burnie bee'. If you want to know the direction the love of your life will be coming from when you meet, set a ladybird on the back of your hand. Puff gently to make it fly away, and watch where it goes, saying:

> *Bless you, bless you burnie bee,*
> *Tell me when my wedding day will be*
> *If it be tomorrow day*
> *Take your wings and fly away,*

Fly to the East, fly to the West,
Fly to him that I love best.

The ladybird will show you the direction your love will come from. No, really!

On a night of the new moon, look at the moon over your right shoulder, take three steps backwards and say:

New moon, new moon, true and bright,
If I am to take a lover, let me dream of him tonight.
If I am to marry far, let me hear a bird cry
If I am to marry near, let me hear a cow low
If I am to marry never, let me hear a hammer knock.

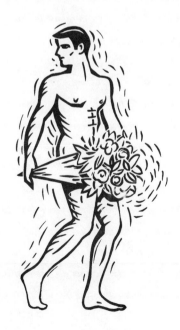

Between The Sheets

MINI FOREPLAY

Each number on the die represents a foreplay listed below.
Each player rolls the die three times. After both players have rolled the die, they perform the allotted foreplays.

1) *Using fragrant oil, draw symbols of love—hearts, suns, stars, flowers—on favourite parts of your lover's body.*

2) *Wash your lover's feet in warm soapy water. Enjoy playing with and tickling each toe; your partner is not allowed to make any noise, and if they do, you can choose the 'punishment'.*

3) *With you naked, make your partner stand perfectly still while you undress them. Play a teasing game with each piece of clothing as you remove it.*

4) *Stroke your naked partner all over with a silk scarf wrapped over your hand or held loosely: between the thighs, over closed eyes, lightly draped over nipples and buttocks . . .*

5) *In the bath, work up a soapy lather on your partner's back. Write secret messages in the lather and let them try to guess what they are. Make your lover pay a price for each answer they can't guess by promising you a favourite sexual treat afterwards.*

6) *Dress up and perform as your lover's favourite fantasy partner: servant, soldier, doctor, teacher . . . use your imagination, but make sure you leave some interesting bits of bare flesh.*

★ ★

Hot Spots
Chilli Almonds

Heat some chilli powder in hot oil in a pan, then sauté some almonds
in the mixture until golden brown. Serve hot!

★ ★

Truth or dare

Answer these with your partner—if you dare . . .

How sexually inhibited are you?

A) Not at all

B) Not very

C) Fairly

D) Very

It's natural to have some hang-ups! 45% of men and 53% of
women say they are very or fairly sexually inhibited.

Truth or dare

Answer these with your partner—if you dare . . .

Which of the following things make you less inhibited in bed?

A) Alcohol

B) An adventurous partner

C) Feeling very aroused

D) Being out of the usual surroundings

A change is as good as a holiday . . . Nearly a third of men
and women get a sexual charge from a change of scene.

I

In what exotic place would you like to make love?

II

Describe how you feel when you have an orgasm.

III

Talk about a current sexual fantasy.

© 1989

Blindfold yourselves and undress each other, touching and caressing each part of the body as it is revealed.

I

Explain how oral sex should be performed on you?

II

Do you enjoy using gadgets in your love making sessions?

III

Do you remember when you first became aware of your sexuality?

© 1989

❋ SENSUAL CLASSICS ❋

Enjoy these surefire musical masterpieces with your lover
as a prelude to passion.

The adagietto from Mahler's Fourth Symphony

Schubert Piano Trio opus 99 (especially the slow movement)

The trio 'Soave il Vento' from Mozart's opera *Cosi Fan Tutti*

The last movement from Tchaikovsky's Fifth Symphony

Johann Strauss' Four Last Songs

Dvorak Piano Trio in E Minor opus 90, 'The Dumky' (especially
the Andante)

Tamino's aria from Act One of Mozart's *The Magic Flute*

Schubert's 'Notturno' D897

Villa-Lobos' 'Bachianas Brasillieras' number 5

Mozart Piano Concerto in C Major K467

Elgar Cello Concerto, played by Jacqueline du Pré

Mozart's Serenade No 10 in B Flat Major (for 13 wind instruments)

Beethoven's 'Moonlight Sonata'

Brahms Piano Concerto in D Minor (the second movement)

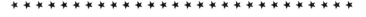

Hot Spots

Serve this Latin lover's sauce with your favourite meats.

Mohlo de Curry
(Curry Sauce)

4 tbsp butter

1 onion, finely chopped

2 tbsp flour

1–3 tbsp curry powder

1 cup beef broth

1 apple, peeled and chopped

$^1/_2$ tsp salt

1 tbsp apple chutney

$^1/_2$ tsp lemon juice

Melt the butter in a saucepan. Add the onion and fry for 5 minutes until golden brown. Stir in the flour and curry powder and cook for 1 minute. Add the beef broth gradually, stirring constantly, and cook until the sauce is smooth. Add the apple and salt. Cover and simmer for 20 minutes.

Stir in the apple chutney and lemon juice and serve hot.

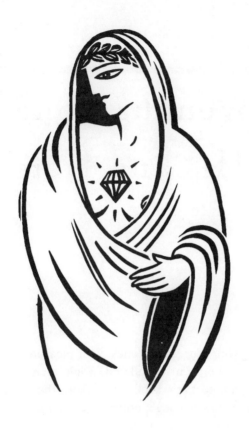

Keep in mind the sensual effects of different fabrics when you have excitement in mind. The feel of your clothes will contribute to the mood. Think:

Leather Fur Silk Velvet Suede Satin
Silk Crisp cotton Lace

Erogenous Zones— His and Hers

Where are your erogenous zones, your pleasure spots? And how do you like them stimulated? Some men like to have attention paid to their backs, especially the small of the back, with a slow massage; others like their nipples played with. A woman may be more turned on by the kissing of her inner thigh, or her feet, than by a concentration on her breasts. For further hints, see Erotic Highlights below.

Getting to know each other physically should be full of delicious surprises. Take it as slowly as you can, so that there is still something left to discover. Using the diagrams on pages 36 and 37, mark in your pleasure spots—where they are and what you like done to them. Show them to your lover and, if these diagrams are inadequate, show your lover what you like in the flesh, using your body as a three-dimensional diagram.

And don't be restricted by what your lover's chart reveals! There may be tricks you know that your lover hasn't thought of. Experiment and explore. All the fun of discovering new sensual horizons awaits you.

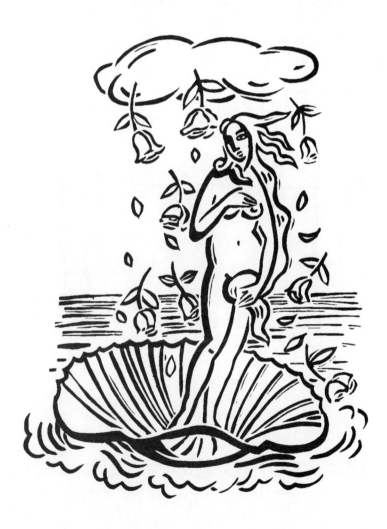

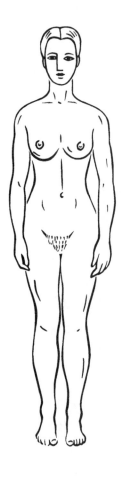
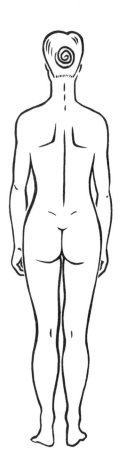

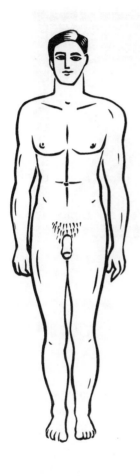
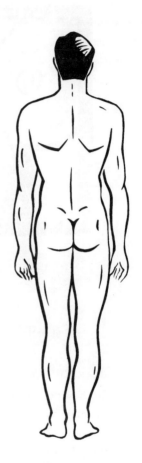

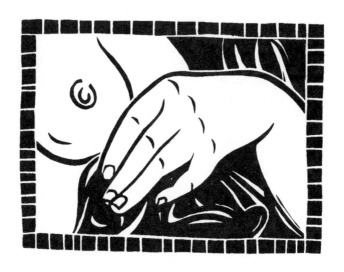

Erotic highlights — hers

BEHIND HER EARS

Both sexes find that the ears are very sexually sensitive, perhaps because they're slightly secret and private. Lots of women love to be stroked, tickled and caressed behind the ears. Gentle kissing can arouse some women: others love their ears licked and lobes sucked.

THE BACK OF HER NECK

The nape of the neck is a highly sexually charged area. Run your lips up her spine to the point where the hair begins.

HER NIPPLES AND BREASTS

These very attractive parts of the body can give enormous pleasure to both parties! The breasts can be cupped, stroked and massaged (but make sure it is not too vigorous). The skin around the nipple, the areola, is amazingly sensitive, and nearly all women enjoy this area being tongued, as well as having the nipples themselves sucked and even tenderly bitten.

HER RIBS

Run your mouth along each rib, kissing as you go, and trace their contours with the tip of your tongue or finger.

HER ARMPITS

These are also private places, and surprisingly attractive! Try kissing, nuzzling and licking these spots. The subtle feminine scents produced in this region of the body can be a real turn-on.

HER WRISTS

Kiss and lightly stroke the inside of the wrist—waves of pleasure and sensual delight will travel all over!

HER NAVEL

Some women allegedly climax simply through having their tummy buttons stimulated. Even if your partner doesn't quite respond this way, she may enjoy having her navel stroked or kissed.

HER BUTTOCKS

The female buttocks are very sensitive areas, which can be stroked, kissed, patted and squeezed with enjoyment on both sides.

THE INSIDES OF HER THIGHS

Leave these until well into your foreplay fun, then lavish them with tickling, kissing, stroking and licking.

THE BACKS OF HER KNEES

Your loved one may respond well to your nibbling and nuzzling the backs of the knees.

THE SOLES OF HER FEET

These are rather private parts, and therefore she may like them stroked and kissed. Watch out if she's ticklish!

HER TOES

Men and women alike are often turned on by a 'toe job'— suck and gently bite each of the toes in a playful way.

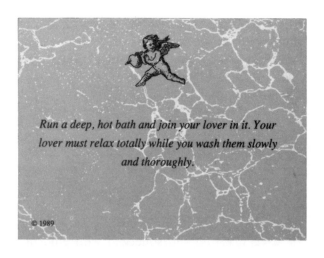

Run a deep, hot bath and join your lover in it. Your lover must relax totally while you wash them slowly and thoroughly.

© 1989

Erotic highlights — his

HIS HAIR

Many men like their hair being ruffled and stroked.

UNDER HIS JAW

Just under the jaw, on either side of the Adam's apple, is a sexually sensitive area. Nuzzle and kiss here for good results.

HIS EARS

Like women, most men find pleasure in having their ears kissed, licked and nuzzled.

HIS BACK MUSCLES

Stroke, massage and gently prod the muscles—this is particularly pleasurable if your man's had a hard day's work.

HIS NIPPLES

The male nipple and the surrounding areola are often ignored, but they are frequently almost as erogenous as women's. Stroking, kissing, gently pinching or nibbling can turn him on.

HIS BUTTOCKS

Lots of sensual nerve endings in this area—it's surprising how many men love having their buttocks played with!

HIS FEET

For a sensual feet treat, see 'toe jobs' above—make sure your partner is a hygienic chap with nice-smelling feet, though!

Stoned on Love

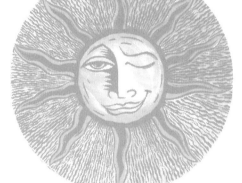

THE POWER OF CRYSTALS

Since ancient times, precious stones and crystals have been given powers of easing or aiding the passions and healing sickness. Gems are given as gifts to mark life events, and there are even different stones for the months of birth, and for each anniversary. Recently, the cult of the crystal has resurfaced, with crystal shops springing up everywhere, offering stones for all purposes. If you want to please your lover with a rare birthday gift, you'll need to know the birthstones for each month.

Birthstones

JANUARY	Garnet
FEBRUARY	Amethyst
MARCH	Aquamarine
APRIL	Diamond
MAY	Emerald
JUNE	Pearl
JULY	Ruby
AUGUST	Sardonyx
SEPTEMBER	Sapphire
OCTOBER	Opal
NOVEMBER	Topaz
DECEMBER	Turquoise

Most of us are attracted to our favourite stones by their colour. But there are other qualities that gems have which you may not know . . .

AMETHYST

The name of this violet or purple variety of quartz is derived from the Greek for 'moderation'. If you wear an amethyst while drinking you won't get drunk or have a hangover—so they say. The stone is also associated with the heart and is said to bring peace of mind and divine love, and to ease heartache.

EMERALD

This bright green beryl has long been considered the 'gemstone of the universe' and has been highly valued since about 2000 BC. It was sought after by the Egyptians in Cleopatra's time, and Roman women wore this jewel in the cleavage to stimulate sexual powers. It has been used for medicinal value, to improve poor eyesight, protect against poisoning, and ensure fertility. Because of these associations, the emerald has been used in rites to incite lust and love.

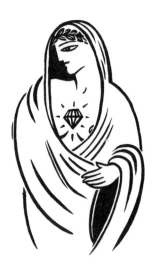

GARNET

The ancient Egyptians adored this stone, and it held its favour until well into the nineteenth century. In the Victorian era it was much in use for bracelets and brooches. The garnet carries strong connotations of friendship, but it also has an affinity with love.

RHODONITE

This stone can range in colour from a brownish pink to a rose-red with black veins running through it. This is another purifying stone, which is known to ease the emotions, reduce stress and calm the mind. Rhodonite will also boost your confidence and self esteem—a good start to any love games.

ROSE QUARTZ

The colour of passion, rose quartz is widely thought of as a love stone. It is believed to ease sexual imbalances and enhance fertility. This beautiful pink quartz is said to boost creativity, invite compassion and inflame passion.

RUBY

Derived from the Latin rubeus—meaning red—the ruby is said to represent the joy in sex. The Hindus revered it as the Lord of Gems, with its regal red glow that would burn steadily to inflame passion.

SAPPHIRE

This stone has always been connected with faith, religion and the mystical world. Devout Buddhists attribute sacred magical powers to the sapphire, while ancient Indian mythology depicts this pretty gemstone as a feminine force, denoting loyalty in love.

TURQUOISE

This stone enhances creative expression, emotional balance and good friendship. It is also said, rather bizarrely, that anyone wearing turquoise will not fall from a horse. If you can't fall off, however, you won't be able to be saved by some passionate stranger! Although the turquoise is a delicate sky blue, the stone also denotes love and passion.

I

What is your favourite time of the day to make love?

II

What is the tastiest part of your lover's body?

III

Should you have long love making sessions more often than "quickies"?

Watch your lover demonstrate how they like to be masturbated.

I

Imagine you are stranded on a beautiful, tropical island with one very attractive person. Describe what happens.

II

What is the latest sexual technique you have discovered which gives you pleasure?

III

Describe what you like best about making love.

© 1989

Oils

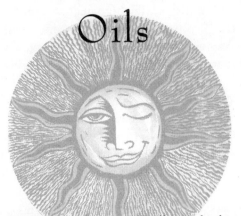

A sensuous massage with aromatic oils sends the pleasure graph right off the scale for both giver and receiver. Not only do you have the thrill of slow, fast, soft and hard touch all over your body, but the scent of the oils can also be extremely arousing.

Experiment with different scents to find which ones appeal most to your lover. A too-heavy or too-exotic fragrance can be a turn-off, so make sure you hit the right note with your partner. You can always try a little blending of different oils, and make your own personal mixture. Here's one to start with:

HAREM CONCOCTION

1 drop ylang-ylang oil

3 drops rose oil

3 drops jasmine oil

1 drop lavender oil

2 drops sandalwood oil

There are other ways, apart from a massage aid, that you can use these suggestive scents. Add a few drops to faded potpourri, or drop some scented oil onto a cotton wool ball and leave it in your underwear drawer or linen cupboard. Oil in a shallow dish somewhere near a warm fire will scent the house. If you have used the same scents in your bedroom games, just walking into this suggestive-smelling environment will arouse your partner and bring a flood of erotic memories.

Don't forget the grassy, herby scents in your search for the right touch. Since ancient times, camomile has been valued for its medicinal properties, and the sweet-smelling perfume can also act as a relaxant . . . imagine that you are stretching out with your lover on a springy camomile lawn. The essential oil from the plant smells like apples and is especially good for the skin. Mint, lemon grass, thyme and ginger are other non-floral scents that could appeal.

The exotic ylang-ylang is a great favourite in South-East Asia, with its scent that combines jasmine and almond. The plant which produces it is a member of the custard-apple family. Try adding a few drops to your bath, or make up this blend for a sexy soak:

BATHING BLEND

3 drops sandalwood oil

1 drop ylang-ylang oil

1 drop lavender oil

1 drop jasmine oil

1 drop rose oil

If you are enjoying a massage, remember that some of these oils can sting if applied to the genital area, so if your massage is going to become more hard-core than relaxing, try the good old standby baby oil instead. You never know, your partner may find the scent of baby oil more exciting than the complex scented oils. Also remember, whether you are using the scented oils or baby oil or even olive oil, that a little goes a long way. A too-slippery massage is not much fun.

Final suggestions: rub each other's naked bodies with oil. Now lie down, and cuddle and wriggle together all over each other. For a more active foreplay treat, a game of naked catch-and-kiss around the house can be a lot of fun with oily bodies slipping just out of grasp! Here's the oil to do it with:

CLEOPATRA'S RUB

3 tbsp almond oil

1 tbsp coconut oil

2 tsp olive oil

1 tsp rose water

1 tsp honey

2 drops basil oil

2 drops rosemary oil

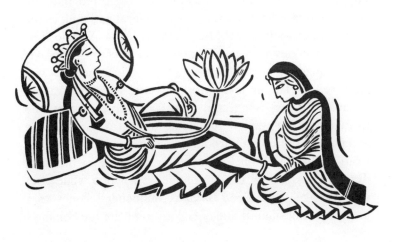

The Nectar of Love

Get the message? The birds and bees have always known about honey as an aphrodisiac and stimulant, and Keats certainly knew about sweet happenings in the dark. Honey was the nectar of the gods on Mount Olympus, and is connected with love and sexuality in many cultures.

Hippocrates, 'the father of medicine', suggested that the ancient Greeks digest honey with ass's meat and milk as the perfect sexual stimulant. Many harems in the Middle East also used honey as a love potion or in sweetmeats. Slavic people mixed honey in cakes as a love potion: the eater was supposed to fall in love with the cake's maker. An old Croatian custom suggested honey be spread over the threshold of the newly weds' home, so that when the bride and groom entered they would merge in a sweet and fruitful relationship. The word 'honeymoon' comes from the early Teutonic tradition of drinking honey-wine for a while after the marriage. The *Kama Sutra* recommended honey as a great source of stamina and energy to stimulate the libido.

Health-wise, honey helps to retain calcium in the body, and is the supreme natural food. Made only by bees and flowers, every part of its simple molecular structure can be assimilated into and used by the body tissues in one hour.

Honey can be a sweet addition to erotic foreplay adventures. Dip your finger in the honey jar and gently caress the luscious amber liquid around your partner's nipple. Or spread it over the body, and with the tip of your tongue explore the liquid on the skin, gently licking and softly sucking it off. Spread it on each other and enjoy a sticky surrender with the scent of honey-flavoured skin adding extra pleasure to a sweet sexual buzz.

> *For he on honey-dew hath fed*
> *And drunk the milk of Paradise.*
>
> Samuel Taylor Coleridge, 'Kubla Khan'

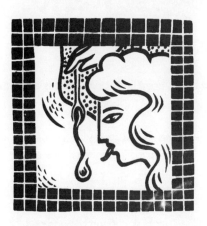

> *You are my honey, honey-suckle*
> *I am the bee.*
>
> Albert Fitz, 'The Honey-Suckle and the Bee'

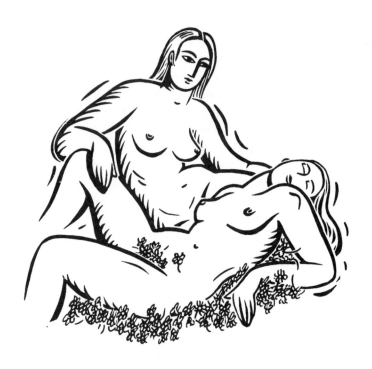

Using a firm brush, paint body-paint designs all over each other's
bodies.

Using your fingers, massage your lover's feet, working
up the legs to the thighs.

Use a creamy lotion to massage your lover's hands.

Think RELAXED to establish a leisurely mood and the mood should
build to sustained passion.

Don't neglect the power of the kiss. Concentrate on the sensation of lip
against lip, tongue against tongue, wet against dry. Suck, lick and bite.

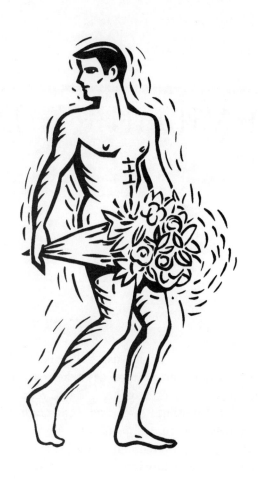

License my roving hands, and let them go
Before, behind, between, above, below.

JOHN DONNE, FROM 'TO HIS MISTRESS GOING TO BED', ELEGY XIX

St Valentine's Day:
Fact and Fiction

For the romantics among us, February 14 is the most important day of the year—a day when all the world can rejoice in a celebration of love. Each year, hundreds of millions of Valentine cards are sent, either signed or anonymously, to the objects of the senders' desire. Thousands of proposals are made and engagements announced, while many more couples walk down the aisle on this day of days.

St Valentine's Day is one of the oldest celebration days, and St Valentine's Day cards, or Valentines as they are more commonly known, are believed to be the first cards ever printed, having developed in the early 1800s from the custom of sending romantic messages. Now there is a dazzling array of cards available for sale, but to show true affection, try making your own—write a poem about your lover and scent the card with your favourite perfume or aftershave.

For lots of people, the sending and receiving of Valentines is simply an excuse for some harmless fun and flattery, for newspaper messages to people called 'Fluffy' from lovers called 'Snookums', but some people take it much more seriously. It's rumoured that when the Chicago gang boss Al Capone learned that his rival bootlegger, 'Bugs' Moran, had intercepted a Valentine meant for him, he was so miffed that he ordered the famous St Valentine's Day Massacre, in which seven unarmed members of Moran's gang were lined up against a wall and gunned down by some of Capone's men disguised as policemen.

There are lots of possible stories behind the origins of St Valentine's Day, mostly related to St Valentine himself (or themselves—there were two of them!). In one story, the Roman Emperor Claudius II, believing single men made better soldiers, banned young men from marrying. Valentine, however, continued to marry couples in secret, so establishing a connection with lovers and the path of true love. In another story, Valentine was much loved by children and, when he was imprisoned, they would toss affectionate messages to him through the bars of his cell window. This may also explain why the sending of written messages has always been associated with the day, although many believe this custom came about much later, as a result of the rhymed love letter written by Charles, Duke of Orleans, to his wife while he was a prisoner of the English following the Battle of Agincourt in 1415.

By the 1700s, St Valentine's Day was well and truly established as a significant day for lovers and a time when partners could be found. One English custom suggested that if a young woman wrote men's names on pieces of paper, rolled each into a small amount of clay and dropped them into water, the first one to bob to the surface would be the name of her future husband. And you thought computer dating was risky!

In another interesting and risky variation, groups of friends met on St Valentine's Day, when each in turn would be given the name of his Valentine. The men would then wear that name on their sleeve for several days. Perhaps this is the origin for the saying 'He's wearing his heart on his sleeve'.

Start planning your own personal Valentine's Day celebrations now. Write down your 'requests' (as intimate and erotic as you dare) and store them for each other in a special box or dish. Then your partner will know exactly what you want—and maybe your wishes will be fulfilled before February 14 comes around again!

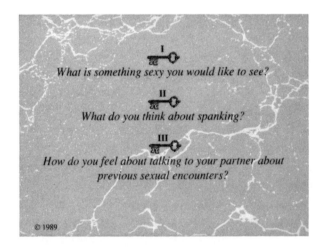

I
What is something sexy you would like to see?

II
What do you think about spanking?

III
How do you feel about talking to your partner about previous sexual encounters?

© 1989

For it was on St Valentine's day,
When every fowl cometh there to choose his mate.

Geoffrey Chaucer, 'The Parliament of Fowls'

Good morrow, friends. St Valentine is past;
Begin these woodbirds but to couple now?

William Shakespeare, *A Midsummer Night's Dream*

Hail Bishop Valentine, whose day this is,
All the air is thy diocese,
And all the chirping choristers
And other birds are thy parishioners . . .

John Donne, marriage song for the wedding of Lady Elizabeth Stuart
and Count Palatine, who were married on Valentine's Day in 1613.

How Does Your Partner Rate
As a Lover?

If you're curious and a little bit brave, try this quiz to see how your partner rates. Turn to page 170 for the score, but if you've rated yourself as a demon lover and your partner as a dishmop, exchange notes—you might be in for a shock.

1. Does your lover have a good foreplay repertoire?
- A)   My lover invented foreplay.
- B)   Yes, but a few more imaginative moves would be good.
- C)   Only if he/she is consulting a sex manual at the time!
- D)   If you count 'Are you awake?' as a turn on.

2. What is your lover's idea of a perfect evening?
- A)   Being the banker in Monopoly.
- B)   Going out with other friends.
- C)   A candlelight dinner and a romantic romp in bed.
- D)   A steamy, speedy seduction when we get home from work.

3. How often does your lover compliment you?
- A)   When I'm dressed up to party.
- B)   All the time, of course!
- C)   When I say 'Do I look alright?'
- D)   Never.

4. *Is your lover affectionate in public?*

    A)   Yes, can't keep his/her hands off me.

    B)   Yes, but it depends on where we are.

    C)   No, we are both very modest.

    D)   No way—we're talking different seat rows at the cinema.

5. *What part of your body is your lover's favourite?*

    A)   Wouldn't have a clue—he/she never tells me.

    B)   Different parts at different times . . .

    C)   All of it, including my nooks and crannies.

    D)   My elbows.

6. *What is the most important part of sex for your lover?*

    A)   Being so close to each other, body and soul.

    B)   The cigarette afterwards.

    C)   Telling friends about it the next day.

    D)   Pleasing me.

7. *Does your lover listen to you?*

    A)   If what I have to say is welcome.

    B)   Yes, of course—all the time.

    C)   Yes, when we're travelling in the car and there's no escape.

    D)   As much as I listen to him/her.

8. *Would your lover be offended if you gave lovemaking directions?*
    A) No. We both give each other directions like 'slower', 'softer', 'harder', 'more'.
    B) No, I don't think so.
    C) We're both a bit too shy.
    D) Yes.

9. *What does your lover think of Saint Valentine's Day?*
    A) A commercial rip-off.
    B) An opportunity for lots of romance and shameless sex.
    C) I sometimes get a token gift.
    D) If I do some heavy reminding close to the date we usually manage to celebrate.

10. *Does your lover still turn you on as much as at the beginning?*
    A) No, the magic has disappeared.
    B) Yes, just as much.
    C) Mostly, but not in the mornings.
    D) Not really, we're not that physical anymore.

11. *Why does your lover love you?*
    A) For my pay packet and connections.
    B) Because together we make a great combo in all departments.
    C) For my body, of course!
    D) I can't begin to imagine.

12. *Could your relationship last without sex?*
    A) No way.
    B) Yes, if we absolutely had to, because there are other ties between us.
    C) Perhaps, I'm not sure.
    D) I think so, but I'd rather not have to test that!

13. *Does your lover ever introduce new tricks into your bedroom?*
    A) Only if I drop a hint with a sex manual left lying around.
    B) Sometimes, but it's such a production.
    C) Yes, all the time: it makes me worry where he/she learnt them!
    D) Sometimes my lover turns on the lights— that's a new trick!

14. *Does your lover lick you in all the places you want?*
    A) No. 'I'm not a puppy-dog' is the reponse if I ask.
    B) Absolutely, and some I'd never thought of.
    C) When begged, and paid back with reciprocal treatment.
    D) I'm too scared to ask.

15. *Does your lover ever make you feel guilty about sex?*
    A) Sometimes, when I'm told I'm too demanding.
    B) No, never.
    C) Often, when I feel we've gone too far.
    D) Yes, I'm made to feel it's shameful.

16. *Does your lover trust you?*
    A)   Absolutely.
    B)   No, I'm closely watched.
    C)   Most of the time, though there are
         sometimes jealous outbursts.
    D)   We've never discussed it.

17. *Does your lover make up quickly after an argument?*
    A)   No, there are sulks for days.
    B)   Only if the argument is followed by frantic
         sex.
    C)   Yes, and we both apologise.
    D)   Arguing would be too much effort.

18. *Which event would your lover most like to share with you?*
    A)   Moonlight bathing.
    B)   Step aerobics.
    C)   Playing pool at the local pub.
    D)   A romantic and sensual evening for two.

19. *Can you talk to your lover about sexual things—really wild stuff?*
    A)   Yes.
    B)   No, most sexual topics are out of bounds.
    C)   I haven't tried.
    D)   Usually, if the mood is right.

20. *Will you still find your lover sexually exciting in old age?*

A)   I hope to find out.

B)   I don't imagine so—I don't want to think about it.

C)   Blek! Are you kidding?

D)   Absolutely, the fires will still be burning.

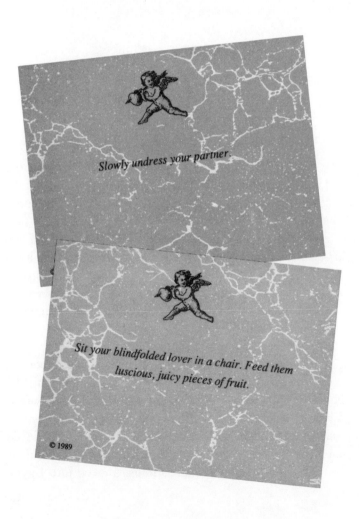

Slowly undress your partner.

Sit your blindfolded lover in a chair. Feed them luscious, juicy pieces of fruit.

© 1989

Stars In Your Eyes

Why is a lovers' walk on a starry starry night so romantic? And is there anybody who doesn't—just occasionally—take a peek at the astrological chart in a newspaper or magazine? When you're caught up in the steamy confusion of a new love affair, the stars can offer some advice. And even if you don't believe in astrology, it's fun to relax with your lover on a lazy Sunday morning and compare the predictions on each other's charts. Maybe your horoscope advises you to go ahead with a new venture—there, you have permission to pursue this affair!

Western astrology has its origins in ancient Mesopotamia, where priests predicted major events by interpreting the actions of their gods, each of which was linked with a planet or star system. As the gods moved, they formed alliances or fought with each other and people believed that likewise the destiny of the earthly nations could be foretold. From Mesopotamia, astrology moved into Egypt, then Greece, where the tradition began of charting the position of the stars at a person's time of birth.

The major elements of a person's chart are their sun sign, their ascendant and their moon. These are defined by which of the twelve houses of the zodiac the sun is in, which constellation is ascending over the horizon, and which house the moon is in at the time of birth. They can determine a person's nature, personality and mental outlook respectively. By establishing these characteristics, astrology can predict how that person relates to others, and which of the other signs are more likely to complement the subject's sign to form a harmonious relationship. And it can also suggest which signs are likely to conflict with each other.

When Shakespeare referred to Romeo and Juliet as 'star-crossed' lovers, he used a widely understood image to show that, as strong as their love for each other was, it couldn't overcome the force of their destiny, or their stars. Right up until the seventeenth century, astrology was a popular science, but, with the evolution of 'modern' science, the old ways fell into disrepute, particularly in England, where they were associated with witchcraft. In today's world, however, astrology has regained much of its popularity.

So, while you and your partner may have stars in your eyes, it could be wise just to check out exactly what stars they are and use the chart on the following pages to see how they match up with each other. Can two perfectionist Virgos live together? How does the stubborn Taurean go with the fiery Scorpio? Now's your chance to find out.

There was a star danced, and under that I was born.

William Shakespeare, *Much Ado About Nothing*

	ARIES	TAURUS	GEMINI
ARIES *March 21 to April 20*	Two competitive rams are great for business, but could be a volatile combination for bedded bliss.		The competitive natures of these signs can create strange but successful bedfellows — Honesty is a strong feature.
TAURUS *April 21 to May 20*	These two can learn from each other. Aries can benefit from Taurus' practicality, while Taurus will discover the thrill of spontaneity.	Routine is the danger here, but both signs delight in indulgence, which should give much pleasure.	
GEMINI *May 21 to June 21*		There's insecurity here, as Gemini's duality plays mind games with the ever-practical Taurus.	The confusion of twins with twins can be some people's ideal fantasy or worst nightmare. However you look at it, it's very complicated!
CANCER *June 22 to July 22*	Great passion can emanate from this couple, thanks mainly to the heat of Aries, but distrust could harm a longer-term relationship.		A good humoured relationship that gets the sexual chemsitry going, although boredom could be a long term problem.
LEO *July 23 to August 22*		A lot of effort has to be made to achieve harmony, but the stability of Taurus can help Leo, and sexual pleasure can run deep.	
VIRGO *August 23 to September 22*	With both parties sharing a desire to please each other, this should be a comfortable relationship.		These two match in some ways, and there should be plenty of passion if they don't irritate each other into separation.
LIBRA *September 23 to October 22*		These two have a tendency to view things differently, but with shared interests they could be able to whip up some passion.	
SCORPIO *October 23 to November 21*	Wow! All sorts of sparks here, but mostly from head-to-head rather than body-to-body interaction. Passion that may just be too hot to handle.		Although there is a degree of common fire and zest (or is it lust?) the intolerance these signs show for each other bodes for a short term affair.
SAGITTARIUS *November 22 to December 20*		If money is the ultimate turn-on, then this is a relationship you can bank on.	
CAPRICORN *December 21 to January 19*	Capricorn may seem too calculating for the free-spirited and impulsive Ram. Not a lot of sexual chemistry here.		The trivial side of capricious Gemini will not be tolerated by the more pragmatic Capricorn.
AQUARIUS *January 20 to February 18*		Sexually, this couple could have some exciting times, but long term plans could make both feel imprisoned.	
PISCES *February 19 to March 20*	Superficially, there appears to be shared benefits here, but it doesn't stand up to close inspection — or a close relationship!		The lack of trust coming from their different natures makes this a relationship that will soon be scaled back.

	CANCER	LEO	VIRGO
ARIES *March 21* *to* *April 20*		Lots of effort needed to achieve harmony. When both signs are willing, lots of passion and pleasure is possible.	
TAURUS *April 21* *to* *May 20*	Mutual understanding can go a long way towards making this a workable relationship, despite Cancer's changeability, which can confuse the bull.		Both enjoy material success: this can provide the trigger for a flamboyant affair which even the tentative Virgo will enjoy.
GEMINI *May 21* *to* *June 21*		Both have quite strong egos, and will not be dominated, even in bed. But with that understood, a lasting and interesting relationship is possible.	
CANCER *June 22* *to* *July 22*	Both are insecure, changeable, and have a tendency to brood over each other's shifts. Nervous tension abounds, but not much romance.		Virgo is a good sounding board for Cancer, and provided he or she can learn to relax, this should be a responsive and durable relationship.
LEO *July 23* *to* *August 22*	Leo's fire is directly opposed to the water of Cancer. It's up to them whether the sexual mix creates heaven or causes joint destruction.	Wow. This really is a great affair. Each simply adores the other, and will enjoy luxuriating in the other's radiance. Hot stuff!	
VIRGO *August 23* *to* *September 22*		There will undoubtedly be a few needlessly cruel barbs between these two, but if they can survive the stings they'll make great bedfellows.	The critical nature of Virgo doesn't go well when mirrored, and all the helpful advice won't make this relationship work any better.
LIBRA *September 23* *to* *October 22*	Libra will be frustrated in trying to analyse Cancer's moods fairly, but more time will be spent on concerns than courtship.		Loads of understanding here, but the relationship will be dull unless something can be found to stoke the fire occasionally.
SCORPIO *October 23* *to* *November 21*		Neither will let their guard down, but there's stacks of firepower here, and plenty of potential for a fiery, if short, affair.	
SAGITTARIUS *November 22* *to* *December 20*	Expansive Sagittarius must spend time making Cancer feel appreciated and needed if the romance is to last.		Sagittarius is just the sign to brighten up Virgo's life, adding the right amount of kindly laughter to generate a spicy love life.
CAPRICORN *December 21* *to* *January 19*		Capricorn is defensive, Leo wary of any competition. The result tends to be silly bickering which takes the fun out of the relationship.	
AQUARIUS *January 20* *to* *February 18*	Creativity abounds, but Cancer may find Aquarius' aloof nature more the basis of a friendship rather than a deeply emotional affair.		Given time, these opposites will attract strongly, and will have a very satisfying sexual relationship once Virgo learns to allow for Aquarius' eccentricity.
PISCES *February 19* *to* *March 20*		Leo will enjoy being the dominant partner, and will rule the relationship with kindness rather than cruelty. A very satisfying relationship for both.	

	LIBRA	SCORPIO	SAGITTARIUS
ARIES *March 21 to April 20*	They say that opposites attract, but beware, the passions aroused in these two can be spoilt by selfishness.		What might start out as a fiery bedroom partnership is likely to fizzle out early in the relationship.
TAURUS *April 21 to May 20*		A dangerously volatile mix, capable of destroying both. Better to back off and accept that some matches were not meant to be.	
GEMINI *May 21 to June 21*	This combination makes for a good friendship, but in the passion department they are somewhat lacking.		A good combination that doesn't get too concerned with things and likes to party — in bed as much as anywhere else!
CANCER *June 22 to July 22*		An intense couple who are in need of some comic relief if they are not to suffocate each other.	
LEO *July 23 to August 22*	Librans will not let Leo dominate, so arguments are likely to result from this combination. A difficult path to walk successfully.		Each is strong willed, and while challenging arguments can be fun for both, there is a danger that the conflict could become too intense. Watch out.
VIRGO *August 23 to September 22*		If sex was all that relationships needed, this couple would get on famously. But there is little understanding, and less depth to the relationship.	
LIBRA *September 23 to October 22*	Librans are possibly the best people to understand other Librans, so this could be the perfect match — provided one can make the first move.		Both these signs are great talkers, and can become close friends, although passion levels may be measured at the low end of the scale.
SCORPIO *October 23 to November 21*	Scorpio's quick wit will outpace methodical Libra, and while Scorpio might enjoy the game, passion will quickly die out as a result.	Lots of fire. lots of friction, but if the times of conflict can be limited, there is also the promise of lots of fun — the sort that knocks your socks off!	
SAGITTARIUS *November 22 to December 20*		Sagittarius may be open and expansive, but Scorpio's ability to play things closer to the chest may result in resentment and hurt. Care needed for a lasting affair.	A good meeting of the minds, and the satisfaction that results can create an equally good and satisfying physical relationship.
CAPRICORN *December 21 to January 19*	A lot of time and effort required to make this relationship work. A tremendous amount of competitiveness to overcome.		A sense of fun can make this a lusty pair who will reach great heights, although a short, passionate affair looks morelikely than a long-term relationship.
AQUARIUS *January 20 to February 18*		This will alternate between hot and cold. Good as a quickie, but woe betide anyone thinking long-term here!	
PISCES *February 19 to March 20*	A soothing association in which there is a great deal of compassion for each other. A good, lasting relationship.		Surprisingly perhaps, these two don't get on. They are deeply suspicious of each other, and ulcers would seem the most likely outcome.

	CAPRICORN	AQUARIUS	PISCES
ARIES *March 21* *to* *April 20*		Both have a passion for adventure and new experiences that will create the basis for an interesting as well as a lasting relationship.	
TAURUS *April 21* *to* *May 20*	These two are likely to make beautiful money together as well as beautiful music. They are a surefire recipe.		An interesting combination of dreams and reality which makes for some varied and very fulfilling sexual encounters.
GEMINI *May 21* *to* *June 21*		Gemini's duality and Aquarius' eccentricity means that there's never a dull day (or night) for these two, even as the years go by.	
CANCER *June 22* *to* *July 22*	This is a good, stable long-term relationship, but the passion is rarely going to reach boiling point.		These two understand each other well, and their deep emotions will create a deep and lasting passion.
LEO *July 23* *to* *August 22*		Both can learn from each other, and the resulting combination will be a passionate relationship that will withstand the test of time.	
VIRGO *August 23* *to* *September 22*	Practicality is the keyword here, and while there is much in common for friendship, there is no magic in this encounter for anything more.		If Virgo can soften its stern approach and bend with Pisces' emotional nature, a very satisfying sexual relationship could blossom.
LIBRA *September 23* *to* *October 22*		Libra's love of perfection may have to be curbed around the absent-minded Aquarian, but the latter may quickly decide there's no point to the exercise.	
SCORPIO *October 23* *to* *November 21*	These are both active signs, and using up energy can make for a lot of fun between the sheets. They can work well together.		These two signs are drawn together by mystical forces, but they definitely need to make actions speak louder than words if they are to go anywhere.
SAGITTARIUS *November 22* *to* *December 20*		These two have a lot in common and can look forward to a long, lasting relationship with plenty of mental and physical stimulation.	
CAPRICORN *December 21* *to* *January 19*	Not a lot of imagination here, and the tendency is for each to apply limits and restrict the other's growth. Not a lot of spark in the sex life, either.		An odd combination that is surprisingly workable, with each benefitting from the other's qualities. The sexual side should also be rewarding.
AQUARIUS *January 20* *to* *February 18*	Aquarius' freedom versus Capricorn's rigidity creates a tense relationship where the waters are seldom likely to run smooth.	The mirror image gives these two a good understanding of each other's unusual ways. Experimentation likely to work more than passion.	
PISCES *February 19* *to* *March 20*		A good balance for each other's extremes sees these signs making lots of hay while the sun shines. A nice mixture of whimsy and creativity.	Their individual fantasy world can create a lot of excitement between the sheets, but there is a danger of both being swept away by the flood.

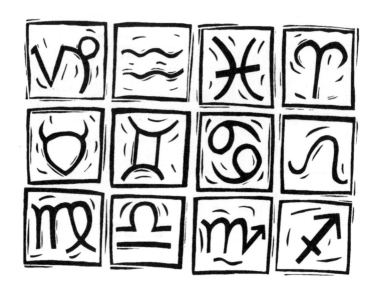

O, thou art fairer than the evening's air
Clad in the beauty of a thousand stars.

Christopher Marlowe, *Doctor Faustus*

Good night? ah! no; the hour is ill
Which severs those it should unite;
Let us remain together still,
Then it will be good night.

Percy Bysshe Shelley, 'Good Night'

*Men always want to be a woman's first love—women like to
be a man's last romance.*

Oscar Wilde

The heart that loves is always young.

Greek proverb

*At such an hour the sinners are still in bed resting up from
their sinning of the night before, so that they will be in good
shape for more sinning a little later on.*

Damon Runyan, 'The Idyll of Miss Sarah Brown'

*Love is the answer, but while you're waiting for the answer,
sex raises some pretty good questions.*

Woody Allen

❁ TEN RAUNCHY MOVIES ❁

*Don't expect to last to the end of these films
without passionate interruptions . . .*

Two Moon Junction

Poison Ivy

Betty Blue

Body Heat

9 1/2 Weeks

Fatal Attraction

Angelheart

Wild Orchid

Basic Instinct

The Hot Spot

Fruit of Paradise

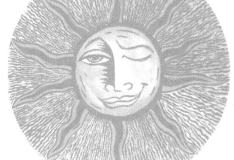

The apple, with its juicy white flesh and ruby red skin, has been the fruit of desire since the beginning of creation. That was when the serpent tempted Adam and Eve in the Garden of Eden . . . 'And the woman saw that the tree was good to eat, and fair to the eye, and delightful to behold; and she took the fruit thereof and did eat and did give to her husband, who did eat.' Eve takes that first bite, the juice runs down her chin and Adam is helplessly seduced. Ever since then the apple has remained a symbol of temptation, seduction, sin—the works!

In Greek mythology, the apple has always been at the core of strife, passion and desire. Eris, a snake-haired, jealous goddess, was left off the guest list of a wedding on Mount Olympus. Storming in like the bad fairy at Sleeping Beauty's christening, she gatecrashed the ceremony and threw down a golden apple addressed 'To The Fairest'. Eris was hoping to create a brawl among the Olympian egos as they all tried to claim the apple. Instead, three contestants were unanimously elected. Hera, statuesque and severely beautiful, was the Queen of Olympus, consort of Zeus. Blue-eyed Athena was the goddess of wisdom, and Aphrodite, the goddess of love and desire.

Paris, the handsomest mortal man, was called to judge which goddess was the most beautiful. All three tried to bribe him: Hera offered power, Athena wisdom, and Aphrodite promised him the most beautiful mortal woman for his wife. Paris awarded the apple to Aphrodite, and with her help he seduced Helen, and won his heart's desire.

Another tantalising tale of love and desire involves the virgin huntress, Atlanta. Aphrodite gave a gift of golden apples to Meilanion, one of Atlanta's suitors. To win her affections, he had to beat her in a foot race: if she caught him, she would slay him . . . He threw the golden apples in Atlanta's path to distract her and prevent her pursuit. Atlanta lost the race (probably on purpose!) and Meilanion claimed her for his own.

The apple is an emblem of love in many Northern European countries. Scandinavian gods kept themselves forever young by eating the golden apples given to them by the goddess Idunn. To be young, of course, is to love, and to make love, so Idunn, like Aphrodite, was doing her bit for foreplay and other fun with her magic apples.

Folklore uses apples as love charms in the search for a mate. Here are just some of the tricks to try:

❤

On Hallowe'en eat an apple in the dark while looking in the mirror and holding a lighted candle. The reflection of your next bedmate will appear in the mirror.

❤

Peel the skin off an apple in one long strip and throw it over your shoulder. The peel should fall in the shape of a letter of the alphabet. This is the initial of your true lust object.

❤

Confused about several potential partners? Take an apple pip for each. Drop the pips one by one in the fire, and for each pip say one of the names. The pip which explodes with a popping sound will be the one . . . and sex with that partner will obviously be explosive.

❤

Cut an apple in half, whispering the name of your desired lover. If you make a clean cut without cutting the pips, that lover will be yours.

❤

Some amorous apple games can be played in public and concluded in private. Bobbing for apples has always been a favourite party trick with the young, and can be part of more adult frolics, too. Fill a very large bowl of water, and float several secretly marked apples in it. Each player tries to grab an apple with the teeth or lips—no hands allowed. Those who manage to secure an apple will pair off with the person who marked that fruit.

❤

Try this fruity icebreaker with a group of people. Hold an apple under the chin, and pass it on to the next person, who grabs it under their chin, all without using hands! In a game where the apple mustn't fall to the ground, a lot of body parts come into contact!

Like an apple tree among the trees of a grove
so is my beloved compared to other men
I love to sit in its shadow
and its fruit is sweet to my taste.

He brought me to his festive hall
and raised the banner of love over me.
Stay me with flagons
and comfort me with apples
for I am faint with love.

Adapted from *The Song of Songs*

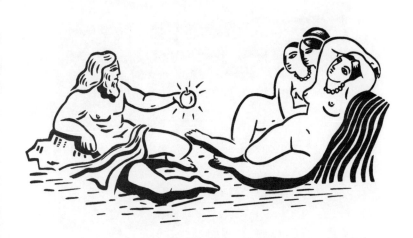

A healthy sex life increases your brainpower! British University research reveals that people who make love at least twice a week are more likely to have a high IQ!

The biggest purchasers of pornographic videos are happily married couples—no, really! About 60% of X-rated video buyers are married and 10% are in a steady relationship.

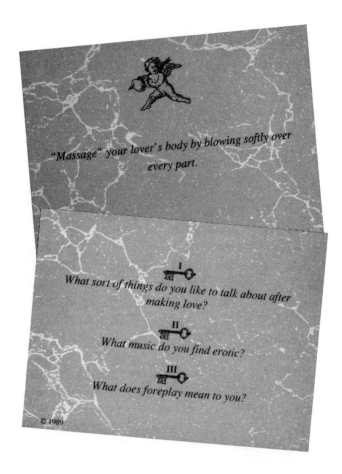

"Massage" your lover's body by blowing softly over every part.

I
What sort of things do you like to talk about after making love?

II
What music do you find erotic?

III
What does foreplay mean to you?

© 1989

Between The Sheets 4
FINISH THE FANTASY 2

Roll the die and the highest score begins. Each number on the die is represented by one of the fantasies below.

Read out whatever number you get on the die and complete the fantasy.

1) *It was a beautiful summer's day and we were having a lovely picnic in a secluded forest . . .*

2) *I thought I was going to end the night quietly at the gym, until I realised I wasn't the only person in the sauna . . .*

3) *I never thought I'd be doing it in my own office, but . . .*

4) *I was asked to join in an orgy. It took a long time to convince me, and a little Dutch courage, but finally I decided to . . .*

5) *The only other person in the lift with me had the most beautiful body I had ever seen. I was just beginning to think how hot the lift was becoming, when there was a sudden jolt, and there we were, just the two of us, stuck . . .*

6) *It started at a Masked Ball, where no one knew exactly who was their partner . . .*

Truth or dare

Answer these with your partner—if you dare . . .

How satisfied are you with your sex life at the moment?

- A)   Very satisfied
- B)   Fairly satisfied
- C)   Not very satisfied
- D)   Not at all satisfied

Looks like we've all got lots of room for improvement. Nearly a quarter of men and women are not very or not at all satisfied with their current sex lives.

Truth or dare

Answer these with your partner—if you dare . . .

Which of the following would you like to do, but feel shy about suggesting?

- A)   Making love in front of a mirror
- B)   Undressing in front of you partner
- C)   Sharing sexual fantasies
- D)   Oral sex
- E)   Asking for something new

Start telling each other what you'd *really* like! 21% of women want to share their sexual fantasies and nearly a quarter of men would like to try oral sex.

Don't underestimate the erotic power of surprise . . .

Why not slip a note in your lover's pocket revealing your favourite fantasy.

Or whisper something dirty in your lover's ear while in public.

The surprise of wearing no underwear can be a big turn-on, especially if your lover discovers this while you are out together (a roving hand finding flesh instead of fabric, a naughty glimpse à la Sharon Stone).

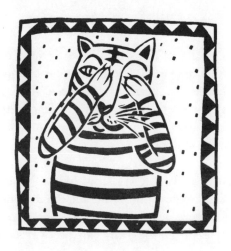

Tropical Tango

THE MOUTHWATERING MANGO

The mango is one of the world's most erotic, exotic, and succulent fruits. Its sweet smell, tangy taste, and sensuous texture makes it the perfect aphrodisiac food, especially when its skin has a tender rosy blush. Mangoes ripen in the summer, that season of warm afternoons, sultry nights, and fewer and fewer clothes.

When a mango feels soft yet firm, like a young woman's breast, it's ready to devour. Try licking the top end of a cool mango as if it were a nipple, then sink your teeth into it. The piquant taste of the skin will be overtaken by the sweet flesh. Slowly pull back the top part of the skin and eat into the rest of the fruit to the stone.

Mangoes are so juicy that a good place to eat them together is in the bath; whether there is water in it or not . . . Annoint each others' bodies with the soft flesh of the mango, exploring all your favourite parts. Let the juice flow into belly-buttons and other nooks and crannies . . . lovely places from which to lick it up.

First cultivated about 4,000 years ago, the mango is indigenous to Burma, the Malay Archipelago and India, where over a hundred varieties are grown. The oval shaped fruit is rich in vitamins A, B, and D, and will help sustain the most torrid of tropical lovemaking sessions.

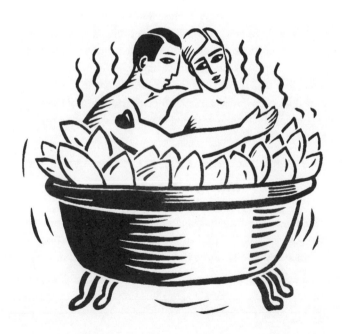

* *

Mango Blossom Mousse

2 medium-sized mangoes, peeled and sliced

2 tbsp caster sugar

1 tbsp gelatine

3 tbsp orange juice

300 ml cream

Garnish

extra cream, whipped

grated chocolate

Puree the mango to make 2 cups. Add the sugar to the pulp and mix well. Sprinkle the gelatine over the orange juice and place over hot water to dissolve. Fold dissolved gelatine and juice through the mango pulp. Whip cream until soft peaks form, then fold through mango mixture. Pour into a bowl or individual mousse dishes, and refrigerate until firm. Decorate with whipped cream and grated chocolate. Ideal served with the coldest possible champagne!

* *

Mango Nectars

Don't forget the fragrant mango daiquiri (see Love Potions). Mangoes can also be used in coladas (instead of banana), or combined with the Japanese Rubis liqueur, cream and milk.

* *

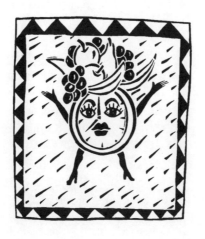

THE PERFECT PAPAYA

The papaya is also part of summer's bounty. The yin/yang of papaya drizzled with lime juice is part of hazy mornings of misbehaviour, when a sensuous breakfast of these fruits makes a return to bed imperative. The scent of papaya conjures up tropical images of Gauguin's works, where luscious Tahitian maidens lounge and strut in their simple and colorful pareos . . . what better unisex clothing for a hot summer than a cotton wrap which can be discarded so easily?

E. J. Banfield, who escaped to a tropical island, believed passionately in the many beneficial properties of the papaya. It is not only delicious to eat, but, if you are a woman, by eating it 'your complexion will become more radiant. If a mere man you will be the manlier.' And we all know what he meant by *that*.

Banfield also tells his readers that papaya leaves wrapped around meat will make it more tender, and that the milk of the snapped branches has medicinal uses. Here he describes his breakfast:

> *'The stalk must be carefully cut, and the spice-exhaling fruit*
> *borne reverently to the table. The rite is to be performed in*
> *the cool of the morning, for this is essentially a breakfast*
> *fruit . . . then when the knife slides into the buff-coloured*
> *flesh, minute colourless globules exude from the facets of the*
> *slices. These glistening beads are emblems of perfection.'*
> CONFESSIONS OF A BEACHCOMBER (1908)

Feed your lover cubes of this beautiful fruit as tiny rewards for sexual treats . . . or lay wafer-thin slices of papaya all over your lover's body and nibble them delicately up.

★ ★

Prawn and Papaya Salad

Combine the sultry freshness of papaya with tempting seafood in this tasty dish, bound to arouse other appetites.

1 papaya, about 1 kg

juice of 1 lemon

juice of 1 orange

³/₄ cup mayonnaise

¹/₄ cup cream

2 tbsp chopped dill

750 g medium-sized cooked prawns, shelled and deveined

freshly ground black pepper

fresh dill sprigs, to garnish

Halve the papaya and scoop out the seeds. Peel and cut the flesh lengthways, into slices. Combine the mayonnaise with the lemon and orange juice to taste. Whip the cream until thickened, and soft peaks form, then gently fold into the mayonnaise mixture with the dill. Arrange the papaya slices and prawns on a serving plate, sprinkle with fresh pepper, then spoon over the mayonnaise and garnish with dill.

For a hot result with this cool salad, choose a warm night, take a rug to lie on and serve out of doors.

★ ★

I

Where is your favourite love making place?

II

Do you enjoy the "69" position as a love making technique?

III

How do you feel about instigating sex?

Take a photo of your lover posing in an erotic position.

I

How much independence do you need in your relationships?

II

How do you feel about hugging and kissing without having sex?

III

Do you have difficulty in just laying back and enjoying your lover's attentions?

© 1989

Greek Gods: Orgies on Olympus

How often have you dreamed about a god or goddess walking through your bedroom door? The heroes of the classical past weren't always ideal lovers, however. Their lives were dominated by all the usual bickerings, lusts, infidelities, jealousies and temporary truces. They quite often fell in love with mortals, too, and that's when the really kinky stuff starts . . . The gods usually carried out their seductions disguised as animals, birds or, in one especially rewarding story, a shower of gold. Here are some of the titillating disguises that the divine beings thought no woman could resist:

DANAE AND THE SHOWER OF GOLD

Danae was the beautiful daughter of the King of Argos. She lived shut up in a bronze tower, hidden away from all possibility of a love life, because of a prophesy that the

King would be killed by his daughter's son. Zeus, looking down from Olympus, fell madly in love with the imprisoned Danae. He disguised himself as 'a shower of gold' (sometimes shown in paintings as a shower of glorious sunlight) and as a result of this unearthly encounter Danae gave birth to Perseus.

EUROPA AND THE BULL

Zeus had a fascination for kings' daughters: this time it was Europa. Disguised as a beautiful bull, he played with Europa so gently that she was completely charmed and climbed on his back to go for a 'ride' . . . The bull ran into the sea, and carried Europa away to Crete, where she gave birth to their children Minos and Rhadamanthus.

LEDA AND THE SWAN

Leda was not only a king's daughter, but the wife of the King of Sparta. Zeus made love to her disguised as a swan, and fathered her daughter Helen, and the twins Castor and

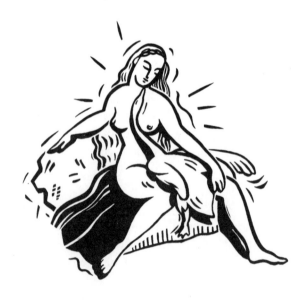

Pollux. The Irish poet W.B. Yeats imagined the seduction scene:

> *A sudden blow: the great wings beating still*
> *Above the staggering girl, her thighs caressed*
> *By the dark webs, her nape caught in his bill,*
> *He holds her helpless breast upon his breast.*

Lusty Zeus had a very busy amorous diary. Inspired by lust, he also appeared as an eagle, a flame, a shepherd, a spotted serpent and a satyr. Perhaps Zeus got tired of being an all-powerful god, but you'd think he would have been more attractive to women as the ruler of Olympus! Perhaps his disguises were to keep his wanderings a secret from Hera, his jealous wife.

Zeus was not the only god to change his form in seeking sexual pleasure. Poseidon changed into a bull, a ram and a dolphin while pursuing various women. Apollo tried sex as a herdsman, a lion and a hawk.

The boys didn't have it all their own way, however. When Zeus turned his lover Io into a heifer to protect her from Hera's jealousy, Hera sent a gadfly to torment Io, and the poor heifer was forced into long wanderings. She ended up in Egypt, where she gave birth to her son Epaphos, and was herself worshipped by the Egyptians as the goddess Isis.

These myths may give you some ideas for divine foreplay games and fantasies. What animal or bird would you choose as your lover? There are plenty of delicious sensations you can enjoy imagining together: the feathery touch of the swan, the creamy bull's soft nuzzling, the strength of the powerful ram . . . Maybe the Greek gods *were* onto something sexy.

Midnight Raids

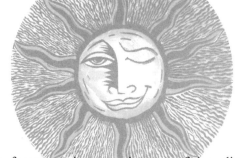

Midnight feasts conjure up images of boarding school scenes, giggling girls making sandwiches in the dead of night. But midnight feasts are also for lovers who want their evenings to last until morning. To sustain your ardour, make sure there are always supplies of quick, delicious and suitably naughty foods in the kitchen cupboards (see our suggestions below).

It's not only the nocturnal nibblies you need to keep in mind. Sometimes a relationship cries out for a whole weekend together indoors, playing sexy games, soaking together in a bubble bath, listening to music by the fire and talking about your deepest secrets and fantasies. Who wants to leave the comforts of bed to go out for food? Plan ahead and your weekend together can be a feast of fine food as well as passion.

Emergency fuel-stops can include easily whipped dishes such as steaming pasta, tangy soups, crisp salads, and indulgent desserts. Tasty morsels both sweet and savoury can be quickly devoured with a glass of champagne to wash them down. For these dishes, stock the following standbys in your pantry:

SAVOURY

Olives, tinned mushrooms, tomatoes and artichokes, capers, dried herbs, ground spices, coconut milk, gherkins, bread-and-butter-cucumbers, chutneys and pickles, harissa, horseradish cream, wasabi, mustard, dry biscuits.

SWEET

Nuts of all sorts (almonds, walnuts, and macadamias to top ice cream, pistachios and peanuts for snacks), chocolate, dried fruit, fancy sweet biscuits.

Fresh ingredients are essential for your amorous culinary adventures. Cheeses, pâté or terrine, sliced meats, eggs, crusty bread, the best fruit and vegetables, fruit juices, yoghurt, cream and ice cream will all serve as love foods.

The first of all considerations is that our meals shall be fun as well as fuel.

Andre Simon

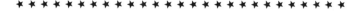

Chocolate lovers

Home-made chocolates are the perfect lover's gift.

Chocolate Truffles

300 g milk chocolate

150 g butter

1 tbsp rum

¼ cup sour cream

60 g chocolate, grated

Break up chocolate and place together with butter and rum into a
2 litre mixing bowl. Cook on high in a microwave for 3 to 4 minutes,
stirring occasionally to melt chocolate. Fold in sour cream.
Pour mixture into a shallow dish. Allow to chill for 1 hour in
refrigerator.
Quickly spoon 1 teaspoon of mixture onto grated chocolate, then
roll it to form a small ball. Coat with extra grated chocolate.
Chill until the truffles have set.

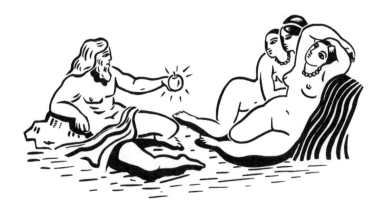

Love Potions

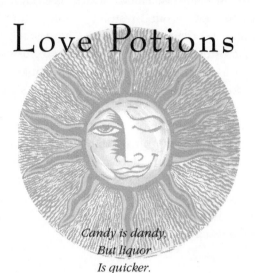

Candy is dandy,
But liquor
Is quicker.

Ogden Nash

From French Kisses to Long Slow Screws and Multiple Orgasms, the names of cocktails hint at exciting things to come. With their vibrant colours and saucy titles, these decadent drinks create a festive feeling whatever the time or place, signalling anything from the beginning of an affair to an intimate evening for longstanding lovers.

Match your cocktails to the seasons. In the summer, whizz up delicious daiquiris from fresh fruit like sensuous strawberries and mouthwatering mangoes . . . In winter, switch to a warmer brew, like the French Kiss, to enjoy together beside an open log fire. Don't forget Alexander Woollcott's fabulous line: 'I must get out of these wet clothes and into a dry martini.'

Over a shared brew of Burning Desire, you might wonder where the cocktail first began. One story says that the word comes from the English racing fraternity around the end of the eighteenth century. Horses which were strong and fast enough to race but weren't thoroughbreds were recognisable by their docked tails. These stuck up like a cock's or rooster's tail, so the mixed-breed horses came to be known as 'cocktails'. As all cocktail drinks are mixed breeds, like the non-thoroughbred horses, it's easy to see how the word-play came about.

Another legend begins in a New England tavern at the time of the American War of Independence. The tavern owner prepared a dish decorated with a rooster's tail feathers. French and American officers toasted the dish with a mixed drink served up by the tavern-keeper, and the story is that Lafayette raised his glass and exclaimed 'Vive le Coq's tail!'

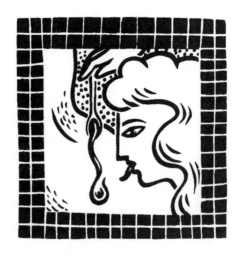

However the word came to be (and the cheeky reference to interesting parts of the human body is probably part of its charm), the cocktail is now connected with the sophisticated high life. Noel Coward introduced sipping in style into his play *The Vortex* in the 1920s, and his later works feature lots of cocktail preparation and drinking. In the world of F. Scott Fitzgerald's *The Great Gatsby*, extravagant cocktail parties were a way of life, while during the Prohibition in the US, cocktails were a clever way of diluting the strong bootleg liquor.

And what about the movies? In *Casablanca*, Rick (Humphrey Bogart) and Ilsa (Ingrid Bergman) start their famous love affair with champagne cocktails in Paris— 'Here's looking at you, kid.' It's followed up years later in Rick's Casablanca bar, where Rick wonders, 'Of all the gin joints in all the towns all over the world, she walks into mine.' Then there's James Bond and his famous martinis, which were always shaken, not stirred; and the fast and flashy barmanship of Tom Cruise and Bryan Brown in *Cocktail*.

Stir up the flames of desire by making some of these exotic brews at home. Put on your favourite music and dress up in evening wear if you have it: tuxedos and slinky evening gowns add a special touch, or even improvise with silk dressing gowns. Let your lover lie back and enjoy being served, or share the preparation of the more complicated drinks, testing some of the indulgent ingredients as you go . . . With the heady scents wafting from lemon peel and fragrant open bottles just waiting to be enjoyed, you may never make it out to dinner.

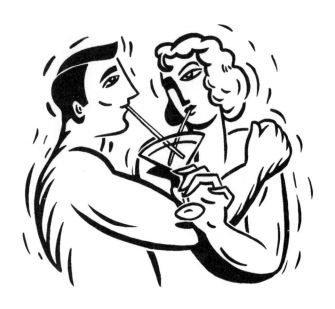

ORGASM

30 ml Bailey's Irish Cream
30 ml Cointreau
Pour over ice in a goblet.

MULTIPLE ORGASM

30 ml Bailey's Irish Cream
30 ml Cointreau
15 ml Amaretto
Pour over ice in a goblet.

BETWEEN THE SHEETS

30 ml brandy

30 ml Cointreau

30 ml Bacardi Light

60 ml lemon juice

dash of egg white

Shake and strain into a champagne glass.

BRANDY KISS

30 ml brandy

30 ml Grand Marnier

30 ml lemon juice

Shake and strain into a cocktail glass.

STRAWBERRY KISS

30 ml Rubis

15 ml Kirsch

15 ml brandy

60 ml orange juice

4 strawberries

Blend until smooth and serve in a champagne glass with a scoop of crushed ice.

French 69

15 ml gin

10 ml Pernod

5 ml lemon juice

5 ml sugar syrup

Pour into a champagne saucer and top with champagne.

Champagne Cocktail

15 ml brandy

15 ml Orange Curacao

2 drops Angostura Bitters

sugar cube

Top up with champagne and stir to dissolve sugar. Serve in a champagne glass.

French Kiss

30 ml Cointreau

30 ml Kahlua

60 ml cream

15 ml Galliano

Mix Cointreau, Kahlua and cream, then top with Galliano. Flame and sprinkle with nutmeg in a champagne glass.

BURNING DESIRE

30 ml Cointreau

15 ml Galliano

5 ml Grenadine

50 ml orange juice

dash of egg white

Shake and strain into a champagne glass.

LONG SLOW SCREW

20 ml gin

20 ml vodka

20 ml Southern Comfort

60 ml orange juice

Shake and strain into a highball glass.

THE LOVERS' COCKTAIL

60 ml Tia Maria

35 ml Tequila

juice of half a lemon

ice

fresh cherries

Stir with ice and strain; garnish each glass with a fresh cherry.

BLACK VELVET

1/2 glass stout

1/2 glass champagne

Pour the stout into a glass. Top with the champagne and stir.

ANGEL'S KISS

25 ml apricot liqueur

10 ml Crème de Cacao

10 ml Crème de Violette

10 ml Prunelle

ice

10 ml fresh cream

Mix the alcoholic ingredients with ice and strain into a tall glass. Float the cream on top.

FOREPLAY

1 tbsp grapefruit juice

chilled champagne

3 tbsp chilled Campari

Mix the grapefruit juice with chilled champagne in a glass. Slowly add the Campari and stir gently.

DAIQUIRI

30 ml Bacardi

15 ml Cointreau

30 ml fresh lemon juice

fruit of your choice: e.g. peeled limes, mangoes, papaya, pineapple

optional: dash of Midori

shaved ice

extra fruit (to use as garnish)

Blend all ingredients in a food processor or blender and serve in a tall glass decorated with the fresh fruit.

CHAMPAGNE COMEDY

Put a small scoop of lemon gelato into a champagne glass and top slowly with champagne.

MIMOSA (OR BUCK'S FIZZ)

½ glass freshly squeezed orange juice

½ glass champagne

Combine juice and champagne in a glass, stir gently.

GREEN AND GOLD

2 tbsp Midori

fresh lime

chilled champagne

Mix the Midori in a glass with a squeeze of lime juice. Top with chilled champagne.

WHITE LADY

60 ml gin

30 ml Cointreau

30 ml lime or lemon juice

Mix together in a jug or shaker over ice. Pour into chilled glasses.

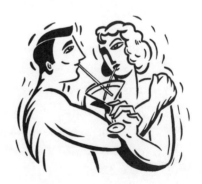

> A little whiskey to make it strong,
>
> A little water to make it weak,
>
> A little lemon to make it sour,
>
> A little sugar to make it sweet.
>
> ANON

MOCKTAILS

If you want the sensual texture, taste and colour of a cocktail without the alcohol, try these health-conscious potions.

TROPICAL TEASER

1 banana

60 ml pineapple juice

60 ml orange and mango juice

3 tsp passionfruit pulp

juice of 1 lemon

Blend all ingredients until smooth. Pour over ice in tall glasses.

SEXY SMOOTHIE

1 banana (or soft fruit such as mango, peach, nectarine)

120 ml chilled milk

5 ml vanilla essence

1 tsp honey

2 tsp yoghurt or ice cream

Blend all ingredients until smooth. Pour into large glasses.

PASSION RISE

50 ml orange juice

15 ml raspberry cordial

50 ml pineapple juice

passionfruit

Shake and strain over ice in an old-fashioned glass.

COCONUT DREAM

60 ml pineapple juice

60 ml orange juice

15 ml coconut cream

1 slice of orange

1 slice of pineapple

4 strawberries

half a banana

half a kiwi fruit

Blend until smooth and serve in a goblet.

LOVERS' CROSSWORD

ACROSS

1. A punishment at school, being ..... may be a pleasure later on. (5)

3. A person with ...... might often be found in front of a mirror. (6)

8. Greek god of love. (4)

9. Before a dinner date, decide who will pick up the ... (3)

11. Wine, roses and music—all very .... (8)

15. Tinkerbell was one. (5)

16. A period of time. (3)

17. Lovers make love whenever they ... (3)

18. Mischievous archer. (5)

20. Lovemaking should involve all your ...... (6)

22. Pleasant smell. (5)

24. Substances used to flavour or scent. (8)

26. A red one symbolises love. (4)

27. Making love can be great ... (3)

28. There was a gunfight at this corral, but it usually means things are fine. (2)

29. Perfume. (5)

31. (and 41 across) Wow! Ooh .. .. (2, 2)

32. .... and pepper. (4)

33. Internal Revenue. (Initials, 2)

34. If unsure, ... (3)

36. A real no-no. (5)

37. Salutes after a banquet. (6)

39. Barbara Cartland is famous for her romantic ...... (6)

41. See 31 across.

42. Opposite of dirty. (5)

43. Present form of to be. She .. (2)

44. Cleopatra's way out. (3)

45. Satan may be, but sex certainly isn't. (4)

46. ..... your lover with chocolates. (5)

48. The song says to 'Stand .. your man'. (2)

50. The grass usually isn't really greener on the ..... side of the fence. (5)

52. Stuck late at night with no money, you may need one of these to replenish wallet or purse. (Initials, 3)

53. Try not to ... on your way to contentment. (3)

55. Short thank you, often used with children. (2)

56. In the past, some cannibal tribes ... their enemies. (3)

57. Happiness is something to ... for. (3)

58. A salty ingredient for a pizza. (7)

59. Nothing more than; only. (4)

DOWN

1. Fondle. (6)

2. The waltz, tango and fandango. (6)

3. This carries blood back to the heart. (4)

4. The path followed by one of 18 across's missiles. (3)

5. (and 25 down) Musical, ... Nanette (2, 2)

6. .. there anybody there? (2)

7. Mae West, the month of May, and ... the Queen of the Fairies. (3)

9. The French say je t'aime or je .'.....(1'5)

10. Males and females have these, although they are usually more prominent on women. (7)

12. Natural form of many metals. (3)

13. The two sexes: ... and woman. (3)

14. An exotic dancer may swing one of these. (6)

15. A tree, not a type of coat. (3)

18. A cool or fancy drink. (8)

19. Fiercely or .... embrace. (12)

21. Arousing the senses or appetites. (7)

23. .... Lisa, a lady with a famous smile. (4)

25. See 5 down.

27. Everyone has a sexual .... (7)

30. Bing Crosby was a .... (7)

35. In the song, it took just one .... (4)

38. A place of revelry more than romance. (6)

40. Cleopatra was said to have travelled in one, although that could just be rubbish. (6)

41. Lips. (5)

42. Priests, men of the ..... (5)

47. Spread made of liver, meat, fish or game. (4)

49. Hamlet queried, 'To .., or not to ...' (2)

51. An ideal Eastern form of activity or conduct. (3)

54. Egyptian Sun god. (2)

56. Present tense of to be, I .. (2)

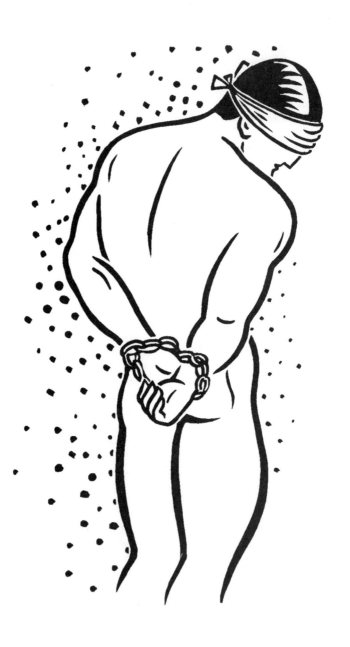

How Confident Are You Sexually?

Are you shy? Are you too pushy? Sexual confidence doesn't always come with experience—some quite inexperienced people have loads of it, while others with a lengthy list of past lovers have none. Think about the people you find sexy, and we'll bet what they have in common is nothing more than a breezy sexual confidence, regardless of looks, income or job. The secret to being sexy is to believe you are. Try our quiz, then turn to page 172 to see how you rate on the sexual confidence scale.

1. *How do you see your body?*
   A) Something to be hidden from the world.
   B) OK, I guess . . . I haven't looked at it lately.
   C) It's not perfect but it suits me just fine.
   D) It's too thin/fat/flabby/bony/dimpled/short/tall.

2. *What do other people think of your body?*
   A) I'm too scared to ask.
   B) Cute and cuddly.
   C) No human has seen it to this day.
   D) They like it, so long as I do.

3. *Do you enjoy making love with the lights on?*
   A) Only on special occasions.
   B) No way, then my partner would see what I really look like.
   C) Yes—on, off, day, night—whatever!
   D) Yes, if I'm sure of my partner.

4. *How would you feel about dressing in kinky clothes?*
   - A) Full of anticipation of some fun.
   - B) Worried about where the candid camera was hidden.
   - C) Keen, but only with the right partner.
   - D) Reluctant: what would my parents think?

5. *Are you sexually jealous?*
   - A) Yes, all the time.
   - B) No, I trust my partner.
   - C) Sometimes, but I try to hide it.
   - D) Frequently.

6. *What is beautiful about your body?*
   - A) I'm not sure, it's pretty average.
   - B) Definitely my . . .
   - C) What isn't?
   - D) Nothing.

7. *Would you masturbate in front of your partner?*
   - A) Yes—wouldn't you?
   - B) Perhaps, but I doubt it.
   - C) Never.
   - D) Yes, but I'd probably have to be drunk.

8. *Do you compliment your lover's body?*
   - A) Yes, both in and out of the bedroom.
   - B) Sometimes.
   - C) Only when we're about to make love.
   - D) No, I'm not that good a liar.

9. *How do you feel about answering these questions?*
   A)   OK, as long as no one sees my answers.
   B)   It's fun, especially doing them together with my lover.
   C)   Embarrassed. Will I be tested at the end?
   D)   Happy enough, though I tell a few lies to stir things up.

10. *What parts of your body would you not let your partner kiss?*
    A)   Anywhere except my mouth and face.
    B)   I don't know, it depends who I'm with.
    C)   My private pink bits.
    D)   None of it—everything's open to exploration.

11. *Did your parents talk about sex when you were a kid?*
    A)   Yes.
    B)   No, only about birds and bees.
    C)   Only once, to tell me too late about the facts of life.
    D)   Yes, but they were a bit shy about it.

12. *Are you able to tell your partner their sexual strengths?*
    A)   What strengths—do you mean snoring?
    B)   Yes, if we've had a particularly good time in bed.
    C)   I'd like to do so more often but it's embarrassing.
    D)   Yes, I can come right out with it any time.

13. Can you 'talk dirty' with your partner?

A)   Yes, we have our own special vocabulary of smut and low-down dirt.

B)   No.

C)   I don't think my partner would approve of the idea.

D)   Sometimes.

14. Has your sex life improved over time?

A)   Not really.

B)   Slowly but surely.

C)   Yes, absolutely, it's always 'on the up'.

D)   I've given up—a book is more satisfying.

15. Do you ever do things that you don't want to do during sex?

A)   No.

B)   As long as it doesn't hurt.

C)   I can be persuaded.

D)   Yes, I'm too scared to say 'no'.

16. Is there anything you would like to do but are afraid to ask for?

A)   Only a few secret fantasies that might get me in trouble!

B)   There's nothing different that I want to do.

C)   No, I always ask straight out—otherwise how would I get it?

D)   I'm afraid of being laughed at.

17. How would you increase the amount of joy in your sex life?

A) I'd read some sex manuals.

B) By letting my sex life evolve naturally, and going where that takes me.

C) I can't begin to imagine.

D) By practising harder and harder at it.

18. Are you likely to make the first overtly sexual move?

A) Not often, but it has been known.

B) Yes, quite often.

C) I'd like to, but fear rejection.

D) No, I'd never do that.

19. Do you change your lovemaking positions much?

A) No, only on public holidays.

B) Not much, I don't want to look ridiculous.

C) Yes, but I need a nudge from my partner.

D) Often, though some I've tried have turned out to be impossible!

20. If you had to find a new partner, would you know how to go about it?

A) Yes, I'd try computer dating.

B) Yellow Pages?

C) I'd go with the flow and wait for something to turn up.

D) Yes, I'd start with singles bars and night clubs.

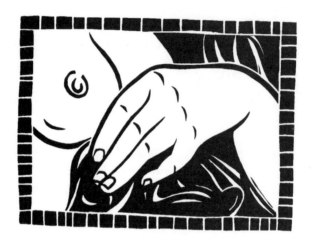

To enjoy the hand as an erogenous zone, try these
delicious tricks:

With your fingertip, lightly trace delicate spirals on your lover's palm, widening the spirals and gradually covering the whole of the hand.

Slowly kiss and suck each fingertip.

Pour a little honey on your partner's palms and lick it up.

With your tongue explore the sensitive flesh between the fingers.

A simple kiss on the palm, French-style, is one of the most romantic gestures.

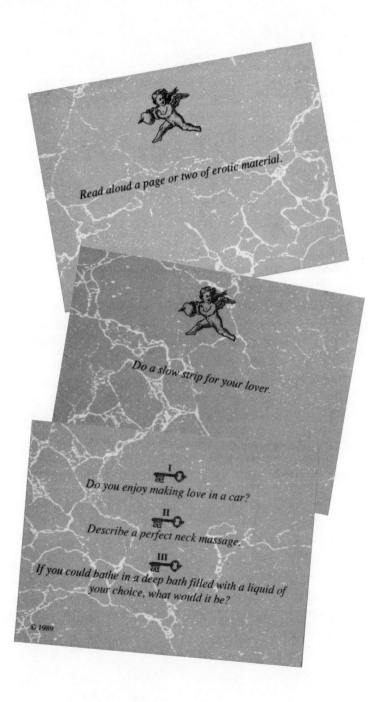

Read aloud a page or two of erotic material.

Do a slow strip for your lover.

I
Do you enjoy making love in a car?

II
Describe a perfect neck massage.

III
If you could bathe in a deep bath filled with a liquid of your choice, what would it be?

© 1989

113

Between The Sheets 2

STRIP DICE

The players each take turn in throwing two dice. Each number on the dice represents an article of clothing, as listed below. The list is a suggestion only, and the players may choose to make their own list, depending on what they are wearing at the time.

As the number is revealed, the partner of the person must take off the particular article of clothing. The winner is the one who gets all the clothing off their partner first. Or is it the one who gets all their own clothing off first? Either way, who cares!

2	Shoes
3	Socks or stockings
4	Underpants
5	Bra
6	Shirt
7	Jumper or jacket
8	Dress or skirt
9	Belt
10	Pants or jeans
11	Tie
12	Watch or jewellery

Hands On

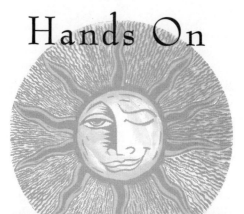

Without the bed her other fair hand was
On the green coverlet, whose perfect white
Showed like an April daisy on the grass,
With pearly sweat, resembling dew of night.

William Shakespeare, *The Rape of Lucrece*

Do you remember the teenage thrill of holding hands for the first time with someone you loved? Holding hands is where many of our love affairs begin, before we progress to more grown-up forms of love play. But even when we move on to a passionate and erotic display of emotion as adults, the hands are still important.

We use our hands, with their sensitive nerve-endings in the fingertips, to touch and caress every part of our partners' bodies, to feel pleasure for ourselves and to give pleasure with our touch.

Hands can also reveal fascinating possibilities about love and sex: how many lovers you might have, how sexually vigorous you are, even whether you have a tendency to infidelity! To find out more about each other—but remember, this is mostly for fun—take your lover's palm and share in the ancient wisdom of these palm charts.

THE MALE HAND

The mind and emotion lines can run together. The heart line with a strong curve away from the head line may show restlessness, or wilfulness in love.

The Mount of the Moon, a fleshy pad near the wrist, signifies romance and fantasy. A flat or undeveloped mount shows a more practical type.

Sometimes the heart line originates from either the head or life line. This can indicate coldness or stunted emotions.

When the heart and head lines blend together, your partner can rely on your impressive physical stamina and a busy sex life.

If the heart line goes straight to the Mount of Saturn, you are a strongly sensual character. 'Platonic love' is not in your dictionary! When the line runs to the Mount of Jupiter, a certain amount of idealism is to be expected in romance, and perhaps some clinging tendencies.

The love line, which falls between Saturn and Jupiter, shows a lover with strong emotions and a balanced approach towards sex.

The thumb shows wisdom and will-power. A strong, flexible thumb which curves back slightly demonstrates a strong character. People who hide their thumbs show little wisdom, and are apprehensive when it comes to declaring their inner feelings.

The marriage lines. If you have one line here you are likely to marry only once. The more lines you have the more times you are likely to marry. If the lines cross, you may be unfaithful in marriage . . .

If you have one full bracelet line then you'll have one major love partner in your life. If two full bracelet lines clearly show, it's likely that you have or will have two love partners at the same time. Now that's something for your partner to watch!

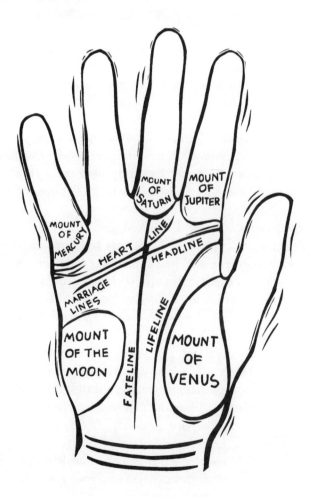

If the Mount of Mercury has a normal size mound, you're likely to be lively, work hard at sex and have a variety of lovers. If the heart line runs over the mound, or is marked by short straight lines, then you are a caring lover.

When the fate line joins the life line at one end and the love line at the other, a strongly independent spirit is indicated.

A rounded Mount of the Moon shows sensitivity and romance. If the Mount of the Moon joins the Mount of Venus, it indicates an extremely passionate nature. If the Mount of the Moon is very high, infidelity could be a habit.

A plump Mount of Venus shows warmth, compassion and sincerity: this person is a good natured and sympathetic lover, mentally astute and intensely physical. A high soft mound could mean inconsistency, while a flat one indicates delicacy, and a tendency to be withdrawn.

If the Mount of Venus is marked with large lines that are crossed diagonally, then you will only have one great love. That love, however, will be strong and everlasting. A lined Mount shows a capacity for strong, long-lasting friendship, coupled with an inability to forgive betrayal. This person is more likely to fall in love with a close spiritual friend than with a stranger.

If you have a Via Lasciva or Milky Way line which curves around the Mount of Venus, you probably take things to excess, from aphrodisiacs to sex, even drugs. A straight line reveals a tendency to boredom. If you have a long curved line then you can be hard to satisfy. And you can also be your own worst enemy!

Two parallel bracelet lines equal a healthy love life. Three lines represent three loves: one young, one wealthy, one happy. If the three lines are deeply marked you have strong stamina for lasting relationships, and for athletic and vigorous sex. Your partner should count their lucky stars!

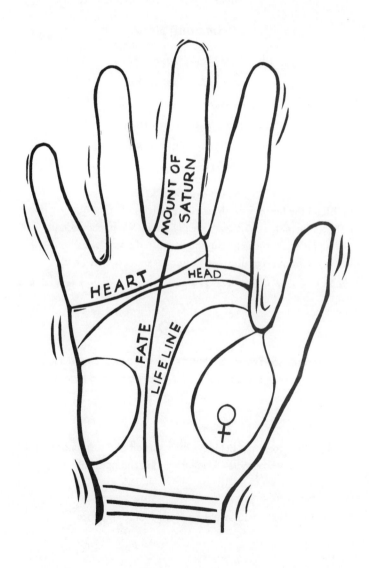

★ ★

Hot Spots

Bring out the devil in your lover with this surefire snack.

Brimstone Bread

250 g butter

10 garlic cloves, crushed

3 red chillies, chopped and seeded

1 tbsp fresh parsley, chopped

1 tbsp fresh chives, chopped

1 French bread stick, cut into diagonal slices

Preheat oven to 200°–250°.
Blend the butter with the garlic, chillies and herbs until creamy.
Spread generously on each slice of bread. Wrap in aluminium foil
and place in the centre of the preheated oven. Leave for 5–10
minutes or until the butter has melted. Serve hot!

★ ★

Flutter a silk scarf over your lover's naked body, then use it to cover
your hand as you stroke your lover. Rub it back and forth between
the thighs.

Take a bath together, but leave the lights off and surround the bath
with candles. Don't forget the champagne!

Flutter your eyelashes over your lover's face.

Teasers

Try your luck at guessing these cheeky picture puzzles. Answers are
written at the foot of the page.

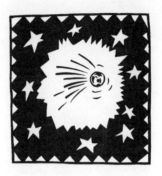

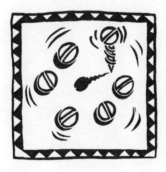

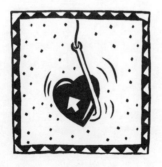

1. the earth moved; 2. screwing around; 3. hooked on love.

Thread flower petals and leaves through your lover's hair. Don't restrict yourself to just the hairs on their head.

Using your tongue, spell out love messages on your partner's back for him or her to interpret.

I
Describe the most intense orgasm you've had.

II
Tell your favourite sexual story.

III
Is there anything you would like to do during love making but don't because you feel it might turn your partner off?

© 1989

Love Food

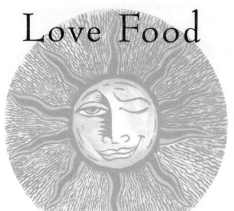

Sharing a meal together, sipping wine, talking and laughing: that's one of life's supreme pleasures, as is wonderful foreplay, of course!

Feeding your lover where there is a bedroom or sofa nearby will inevitably lead to erotic antics, so one of the main points to remember is that the food you serve mustn't be too heavy. Deliciously light, quick to prepare, energy-giving and titillating is the aim.

Let's not ignore the old clichéd seduction menu of oysters and a steak. You don't need recipes for this, just make sure that the oysters are fresh and freshly opened. Serve with lemon wedges and thin brown bread and butter sandwiches cut into triangles. The steak should be a thick cut of the best eye fillet, beautifully grilled. What you don't want is a huge raggedy cut of meat sprawling all over the plate. Potatoes baked in their jackets in the oven will allow you to give all your attention to the grilling, and a leafy green salad can be prepared in advance to await its vinaigrette dressing.

While we're considering such old-fashioned stand-bys, how about thin lacy crepes for dessert? Buy a crepe pan and get someone to give you lessons if you don't know how to do these.

Here's the mixture:

★ ★

Easy crepes

1 cup plain flour

2 eggs

pinch of salt

120 ml milk

120 ml water

15 g melted butter

Whizz flour, eggs and salt in a food processor. Add milk and water gradually, continuing to process until you have a smooth mixture.

Leave the mixture to rest for at least an hour and add melted butter to the mixture just before cooking. Cooking the crepes is easiest if the mixture is in a jug and you can just pour it into your crepe pan.

Cook crepes one at a time, pouring the mixture evenly into the crepe pan, and eat immediately. Sprinkle with sugar, squeeze lemon juice over, roll up the crepe and drizzle with cream or ice cream.

★ ★

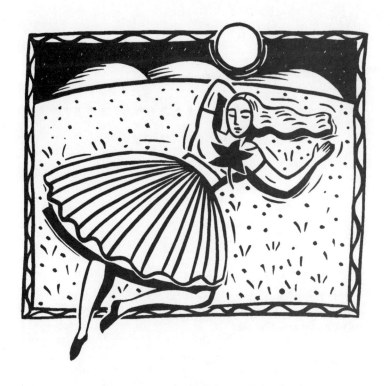

If your relationship is quite new, it helps the 'getting-to-know-you' phase if the two of you prepare a meal together, one as cook and the other as assistant. There's all that brushing-up against each other as you are getting the food ready and sipping your champagne.

If you are longer-term partners, there's probably more of a thrill in one of you (the one who doesn't usually cook, perhaps!) waiting hand and foot on the other.

Here are some seductive menus to try out. It's not necessary to always have three courses, although if you decide to skip dessert it's a good idea to have tempting chocolate or something sweet available with the coffee.

Menu One

Chicken satay

Berries and ice cream

★ ★

Chicken satay

peanut sauce

bamboo skewers

chicken breasts (1 per person)

coconut milk

To make the peanut sauce:
This will keep for weeks in a screw-top jar in the refrigerator. When required for satays, add coconut milk to as much peanut sauce as you will need.

7 tbsp peanut oil

1 tsp crushed garlic or dried garlic flakes

2 tbsp dried onion flakes

4 chillies, seeded and chopped

1 teaspoon dried shrimp paste (trasi)

1 tbsp lemon juice

1 tbsp dark soy sauce

375 g crunchy peanut butter

Heat oil in a pan. Fry garlic, onion and chillies, and remove to drain on kitchen paper. Fry the trasi, crushing it with the back of a spoon. Add the lemon juice and soy sauce.

Remove from heat, add the peanut butter and stir until blended. When cool, add the garlic, onion and chillies.

Mix thoroughly and store in a screw-top jar in the refrigerator until needed.

TO MAKE THE SATAYS:

Pre-soak the bamboo skewers in water. This stops them from burning during the cooking.

Cut chicken breasts into small pieces, suitable for threading onto skewers.

In a bowl, combine peanut sauce and coconut milk, adding 3 parts coconut milk to 1 part peanut sauce. Place chicken pieces in this mixture, and marinate for 2 hours.

Thread meat onto skewers and grill, brushing with more sauce if required.

Serve with boiled rice.

✷ ✷

Berries and ice cream

any superior commercial brand of ice cream (such as Sara Lee or

Norgen-Vaaz)

seductive berries of your choice (strawberries, raspberries, blueberries, etc.)

Dole out generous lashings of ice cream in bowls and sprinkle berries on it.

(For an extra touch, drizzle Grand Marnier over the ice cream and berries.)

✷ ✷

Menu two

Spaghetti with peas and ham
Chocolate and almond cake

★ ★

Spaghetti with peas and ham

(Don't attempt this dish unless you can get very fresh peas.)

1 small onion, chopped

butter

very fresh shelled baby peas, about a large handful each

1 tsbp boiling water from the kettle

ham, about 2 slices each, thinly sliced and cut into matchsticks

cream

spaghetti

In a pan, gently cook the onion in the butter so that it softens without browning. Put in the peas and add the boiling water. Cook for about 5 minutes.

Add the ham and cook till it has heated through. Add enough cream to make the sauce coat the pasta. Heat gently.

Serve the sauce over cooked and drained spaghetti.

★ ★

★ ★

Chocolate and almond cake

This cake has no flour, and is quite rich so you'll only need a teeny slice.

1 tbsp rum or brandy

1 tbsp black coffee

125 g bitter cooking chocolate

90 g caster sugar

90 g butter

90 g ground almonds

3 eggs, separated

In a saucepan, combine the rum or brandy and the coffee. Melt the chocolate very gently in the rum mixture, stirring well. Add the sugar, butter and almonds. Stir over low heat until blended.

Remove from heat, stir in 3 well-beaten egg yolks. Fold in 3 stiffly beaten egg whites.

Pour mixture into a tart tin with a removable base. Cook in an oven at 150° for 45 minutes.

When cool, remove cake gently from tin. Be careful—the top of the cake is liable to crack like meringue.

Top with whipped cream.

★ ★

Menu Three

Roasted tomato salad with crusty bread

Marinated prawns

Fresh fruit

* *

Roasted tomato salad

2 or 3 large tomatoes, peeled

salt

freshly ground black pepper

2 cloves garlic, finely chopped

extra virgin olive oil

basil leaves

crusty bread (enough to mop up the juices)

To garnish:

basil leaves

black olives

For the dressing:

2 tbsp extra virgin olive oil

2 tbsp balsamic vinegar

To peel tomatoes:

Place tomatoes in a bowl, and pour boiling water over them. Leave for 1 minute. When cool, peel off the skins (this should now be fairly easy).

Cut each peeled tomato in half and place in a shallow roasting dish, cut side uppermost. Season with salt and pepper. Sprinkle the garlic on the tomatoes, and then add a few drops of olive oil to each tomato. Top each tomato with half a basil leaf, turning each leaf over to get a coating of oil on both sides.

Place the dish in the oven and roast the tomatoes at 200° for about 50 minutes or until the edges are slightly blackened. Remove tomatoes from the oven and allow to cool. (This roasting can be done several hours ahead.)

To serve, transfer the tomatoes to individual plates. Garnish with basil leaves and black olives.

To make the dressing, whisk the olive oil and balsamic vinegar together and drizzle over the tomatoes.

Serve with crusty bread.

★ ★

Marinated prawns

Enough green prawns for two

Marinade one: mix together olive oil, lots of chopped parsley, lemon juice, garlic

Marinade two: mix together olive oil, soy sauce, ginger, garlic

Marinate prawns in your choice of mixture for at least 2 hours. Turn prawns in mixture from time to time.

When they are ready to cook, throw the prawns into a big, very hot pan or onto a very hot barbecue hotplate. Stir them around until cooked (about 3–5 minutes), and serve.

There should still be some of the crusty bread left from the tomato dish to finish off with the prawns.

★ ★

Fresh fruit

For a tingling variation with fresh fruit, slice an assortment of fruits, sprinkle with icing sugar and drizzle champagne over.

★ ★

Menu Four

Beef and snow peas

Simple pudding

★ ★

Beef and snow peas

Mixture One:

1 tsp soy sauce

1 tbsp dry sherry

2 tsp cornflour

Mixture Two:

2 tsp oyster sauce

$\frac{1}{2}$ tsp sugar

$\frac{1}{2}$ tsp sesame oil

$\frac{1}{2}$ tsp soy sauce

1 tsp Green Ginger Wine

250 g beef fillet, thinly sliced

$\frac{1}{2}$ cup oil

pinch of salt

extra 2 tbsp oil

250 g snow peas

$\frac{1}{2}$ tsp cornflour mixed with 1 tbsp water.

Marinate beef for 15 minutes in Mixture One.

Heat oil and fry beef until brown. Remove and set aside.

Add salt to the extra oil, heat, and sauté snow peas until bright green.

Return beef to pan and add Mixture Two. Add the cornflour mixed with water, blend and serve immediately.

★ ★

Simple pudding

Amaretti biscuits

any sweet Italian liqueur, or a sticky dessert wine

mascarpone

Pile some Amaretti biscuits into a pretty bowl.

Give each person a glass of the liqueur or wine, and a dish containing a dollop of mascarpone.

Take a biscuit, dunk it in the wine in the glass, then scoop up some mascarpone with the biscuit and enjoy.

The wine is to be sipped as well, of course!

★ ★

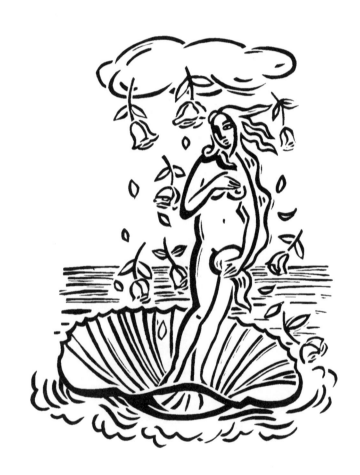

I

Do you find it easy to show affection?

II

How do you feel about making love in a lift that you've stopped between floors?

III

Discuss a wonderful time you remember sharing together.

Place a large sheet of plastic on the floor. Cover your body and your lover's body with oil and have a wrestling match on the plastic.

I

What was the most romantic love making session you've ever experienced?

II

What is your best physical attribute?

III

Talk about something erotic you'd like to do with a piece of fruit.

Between The Sheets 8
MINI FOREPLAY

*Each number on the die represents a foreplay listed below.
Each player rolls the die three times. After both players have
rolled the die they perform the allotted foreplays.*

1) Have an assortment of feathers ready and brush, stroke
   and tickle your partner's body with them. Find out which
   are the most responsive parts, and then swap so your
   lover does the same for you.

2) Dust talcum powder all over your partner's body. Take
   an ice cube and use it to make patterns through the
   powder. The feeling of cold on hot skin is sensational.

3) Make a list of sexy ideas and whisper them into your
   lover's ear. Ask him/her to rate the ideas from 1–10
   depending on how excited they become.

4) Use a vibrator to massage your partner's body, except for
   genitals and nipples. Avoid these carefully and your lover
   will go wild!

5) After a shower together, use a soft brush and vigorously
   rub your partner's feet, one foot at a time.

6) Relax naked next to your partner for a few minutes and
   listen to each other's heartbeat and breathing.

★ ★

Hot Spots

Bring out the devil in your lover with this surefire snack.

Lucifer's Pizza

1 pizza base

2 tsp olive oil

1 cup ripe tomatoes, pureed

1 cup black olives, pitted

8 fresh red chillies

chunks of fresh bocconcini cheese

Brush the pizza base with olive oil and spread with the tomato.
Scatter the olives, chillies and cheese over the top. Bake in a very
hot oven for about 10 minutes (or until the edges of the base are
brown). Serve hot!

★ ★

—⌒

Lick the *corners* of each other's mouths: these are highly
erogenous areas.

Play fantasy dress-ups for each other. Try roles like teacher,
student, nurse, captor and prisoner.

Undress slowly for your lover. Ask for help with
zips and fastenings.

Flutter a silk scarf over your lover's naked body, then use it to
cover your hand as you stroke your lover. Rub it back and forth
between the thighs.

LOVERS' LITTLE CROSSWORD

ACROSS

1. Sweet exotic tropical fruit. (5)

6. Truman ......, American novelist. (6)

11. Opposite of bad. (4)

12. A space between. (3)

13. This bear could double as enticing lingerie. (5)

14. Bo Derek found this music arousing. (6)

16. As good .. gold. (2)

17. Russian male name, a variant of which was used by one of the men from UNCLE. (4)

18. This in the hair may be hard to see, but still needs drastic treatment. (3)

19. A place to see animals. (3)

22. The mathematical value used in calculations pertaining to circles. (2)

23. In the song, the little girl was told to '.. away'. (2)

25. A romance could be called an ...... of the heart. (6)

28. Engineering Corps. (Initials, 2)

29. A night ... keeps late hours. (3)

31. Is this form of sex safe? (4)

32. Closer. (6)

34. He is, they are, I .. (2)

37. ... fingers and ... toes. (3)

38. French word for love. (5)

39. Pocket originally for a watch. (3)

42. He flew too high and paid the price. (6)

43. Sufficient. (6)

44. Short story or piece of prose. (5)

45. Tranquil Eastern philosophy. (3)

46. Employ. (3)

35. Rolling stones don't gather any of this. (4)

36. Every lover ..... for a night of passion. (5)

38. Greek god of war. (4)

39. Turkish headgear. (3)

40. ... is the loneliest number. (3)

41. Have a good trip! ... Voyage! (3)

DOWN

2. Life was tough in the Dark .... (4)

3. A ... is as good as a wink to a blind man. (3)

4. This lady really rode bareback. (6)

5. A force once held to pervade all nature. (4)

7. 'A long time ..., in a galaxy far, far away.' (3)

8. Buddy. (3)

9. Truthful, honest. (4)

10. Sexually stimulating. (6)

13. It takes two for this one. (5)

14. Eastern market, sounds like it's strange. (6)

15. To mature. (5)

20. Fragrant ..., often used in lovemaking. (3)

21. Either/.. (2)

24. Possess. (3)

26. Alien, strange. (7)

27. A well-known kissing method. (6)

30. French seaport, .. Havre. (2)

33. In, on or near. (2)

34. To entertain, humour. (5)

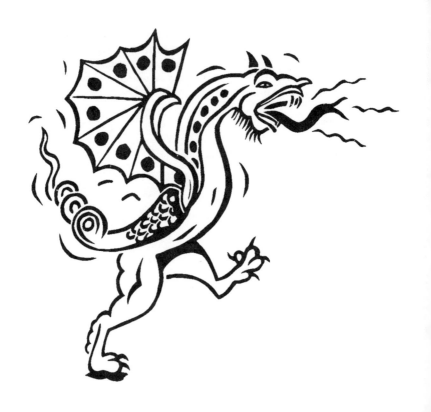

Chinese Astrology

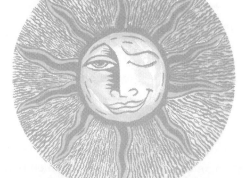

THE STARS THROUGH DIFFERENT EYES

Are you a Rat? Don't laugh, in Chinese astrology, the Rat is a sociable, friendly person, who'll spend lots on the one they love. Perhaps you're lucky enough to have a Tiger for a partner: warm-hearted and sympathetic, a sexual dare-devil. If you're a Dragon—extremely strong, with immense energy and enthusiasm—you might just get on with a Monkey!

We can learn a lot about our lovers through the exotic craft of Chinese astrology, which represents the earliest written records of divination or fortune-telling through reading the heavens. In the Chinese system, it is not the movement of stars which is the key element, but the effect of the sun and moon on the seasons, on life, and on people.

In the twelve-year cycle, each year is represented by an animal. The principle is that an individual is influenced by the characteristics of the year in which they are born. However, there's much more to the eastern system than just the animal year. A key element of all eastern philosophy is the concept of yin and yang: the inter-relationship of the positive and negative aspects of reality. There's no association of positive with good and negative with evil, they're simply the two essential building blocks of the universe. Yin is the negative, feminine aspect and yang the positive, male aspect.

The Rat, Tiger, Dragon, Horse, Monkey and Dog are linked with yang (positive) while the Ox, Rabbit, Snake, Sheep, Rooster and Boar are linked with yin (negative).

The five elements—Metal, Fire, Earth, Wood and Water—represent qualities of mind, a little like Western astrology's four elements of Earth, Fire, Water and Air. Each of these elements has a negative and a positive side, so there are ten element classifications, each of which is also assigned to a year. In other words, each year has both an animal and an element associated with it, but, because the animal cycle is twelve years and the element cycle ten years, the same animal does not always have the same element associated with it. Confusing! In fact, the same animal/element combination repeats only once every sixty years.

The months of the year and the hours of the day are also given the characteristics of the twelve animal symbols. However, for general purposes, it's enough to know the year of your birth, remembering that in the Chinese calendar the year is strictly aligned to the lunar cycle, and New Year falls on a different day each year. We've included a chart to give you the animal/element signs for each year from 1940 to 1980.

For a romantic and amusing evening, invite some friends around, and, over some tasty Chinese food, work out each other's animal and element signs. Then you'll have fun looking at each other's characteristics and compatibility—but don't swap partners on the strength of it!

Feb 8, 1940–Jan 26, 1941	Dragon	Metal	(+)
Jan 27, 1941–Feb 14, 1942	Snake	Metal	(−)
Feb 15, 1942–Feb 4, 1943	Horse	Water	(+)
Feb 5, 1943–Jan 24, 1944	Sheep	Water	(−)
Jan 25, 1944–Feb 12, 1945	Monkey	Wood	(+)
Feb 13, 1945–Feb 1, 1946	Rooster	Wood	(−)
Feb 2, 1946–Jan 21, 1947	Dog	Fire	(+)
Jan 22, 1947–Feb 9, 1948	Boar	Fire	(−)
Feb 10, 1948–Jan 28, 1949	Rat	Earth	(+)
Jan 29, 1949–Feb 16, 1950	Ox	Earth	(−)
Feb 17, 1950–Feb 5, 1951	Tiger	Metal	(+)
Feb 6, 1951–Jan 26, 1952	Rabbit	Metal	(−)
Jan 27, 1952–Feb 13, 1953	Dragon	Water	(+)
Feb 14, 1953–Feb 2, 1954	Snake	Water	(−)
Feb 3, 1954–Jan 23, 1955	Horse	Wood	(+)
Jan 24, 1955–Feb 11, 1956	Sheep	Wood	(−)
Feb 12, 1956–Jan 30, 1957	Monkey	Fire	(+)
Jan 31, 1957–Feb 17, 1958	Rooster	Fire	(−)
Feb 18, 1958–Feb 7, 1959	Dog	Earth	(+)
Feb 8, 1959–Jan 27, 1960	Boar	Earth	(−)
Jan 28, 1960–Feb 14, 1961	Rat	Metal	(+)
Feb 15, 1961–Feb 4, 1962	Ox	Metal	(−)
Feb 5, 1962–Jan 24, 1963	Tiger	Water	(+)
Jan 25, 1963–Feb 12, 1964	Rabbit	Water	(−)
Feb 13, 1964–Feb 1, 1965	Dragon	Wood	(+)
Feb 2, 1965–Jan 20, 1966	Snake	Wood	(−)
Jan 21, 1966–Feb 8, 1967	Horse	Fire	(+)

Feb 9, 1967–Jan 29, 1968	Sheep	Fire	(–)
Jan 30, 1968–Feb 16, 1969	Monkey	Earth	(+)
Feb 17, 1969–Feb 5, 1970	Rooster	Earth	(–)
Feb 6, 1970–Jan 26, 1971	Dog	Metal	(+)
Jan 27, 1971–Jan 15, 1972	Boar	Metal	(–)
Jan 16, 1972–Feb 2, 1973	Rat	Water	(+)
Feb 3, 1973–Jan 22, 1974	Ox	Water	(–)
Jan 23, 1974–Feb 10, 1975	Tiger	Wood	(+)
Feb 11, 1975–Jan 30, 1976	Rabbit	Wood	(–)
Jan 31, 1976–Feb 17, 1977	Dragon	Fire	(+)
Feb 18, 1977–Feb 6, 1978	Snake	Fire	(–)
Feb 7, 1978–Jan 27, 1979	Horse	Earth	(+)
Jan 28, 1979–Feb 15, 1980	Sheep	Earth	(–)

THE ANIMAL SYMBOLS

THE RAT

The Rat is generally an industrious person, with a healthy amount of ambition, who is sociable and has a good many friends. Rats are very thrifty, but there is a danger of this thriftyness crossing the line into stinginess. Others may find it hard to penetrate the Rat's facade, as he or she hides their emotions well—but that doesn't mean they are not romantic or do not have feelings. They do, they simply find it difficult expressing their feelings, and you may have to look at more subtle signs. If a Rat spends money, lots of money on someone, you can bet he or she is in love, even if they don't say it!

Compatibility: Rats are most likely to have a successful relationship with a Monkey or Dragon, while relationships with mature Dogs or Tigers are fraught with difficulty. A young puppy Dog, however, will keep the older Rat very happy.

The Ox

Steadfast, loyal and with a capacity for uncomplaining hard work, the Ox is also strong in his or her beliefs, from which there will be no budging. The Ox makes steady progress without usually displaying great flair or brilliance, but don't be fooled—the Ox is very intelligent and will usually end up at the top. The Ox is conservative and traditional in outlook, and although unlikely to set the sparks flying with a sudden romance, the Ox is deeply passionate; as a relationship builds, the partner of an Ox can look forward to some surprising fireworks.

Compatibility: The Ox doesn't fit well with the Tiger, the Dog or another Ox, and should not even contemplate a relationship with a Sheep—there is absolutely nothing in common between them! Although the Ox gets on well with most other signs, the Rooster and the Snake usually make the best partners.

The Tiger

Despite a reputation for savagery, the Tiger is actually a warm-hearted and sympathetic character, who loves life and likes helping others find enjoyment. They are also usually eager dare-devils who can be a source of delight and amusement, at least for short periods. The recklessness and selfishness that can be so endearing can also be draining over a period of time, but it's worth being round a Tiger, even if it's just in the hope that some of their luck will rub off on you. In love matters, Tigers are extremely emotional with strong sexual drives, so if you want a madcap romance, try grabbing one by the tail.

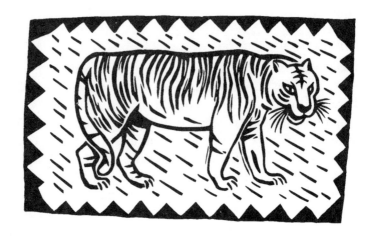

Compatibility: Tigers will get on with anyone for a short time, and they will have some wild flings. For a lasting relationship, they should look to the Dog, Horse, Boar and Dragon, avoid the Rabbit, and steer well clear of the Monkey.

THE RABBIT

The Rabbit is incredibly lucky, and is able to survive adversity better than most. Rabbits are naturally very sensitive, peace-loving people, who quite often display a deep artistic streak. In avoiding conflict, the Rabbit can sometimes appear devious in negotiations, but only for the sake of peace. Despite being understanding of others' needs, the Rabbit can sometimes suffer from disconcerting mood shifts. Rabbits definitely do enjoy the physical side of life—comfort, pleasure and sex—and sometimes their decisions are made solely on the basis of pleasure.

Compatibility: Rabbits form excellent partnerships with the Boar or the Sheep, and can usually look forward to a more than satisfactory relationship with a Dog. They should beware of the Tiger, Monkey and Horse and be especially careful when contemplating a relationship with a Rooster.

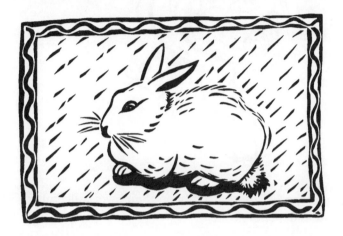

THE DRAGON

In pre-revolutionary China, the Dragon was the symbol of power of the Emperor and mandarins: this animal symbol is extremely strong, has immense energy and enthusiasm, and can inspire others to follow in its path. The Dragon enjoys power, and is often an extremely effective orator, usually at the expense of its enemies. While the Dragon is a formidable enemy, he or she can also be a wonderful friend, helpful and considerate, provided it is understood just who is the boss (the Dragon!). Dragons don't have much energy for romance, and will either form stable if unspectacular relationships while still quite young, or else

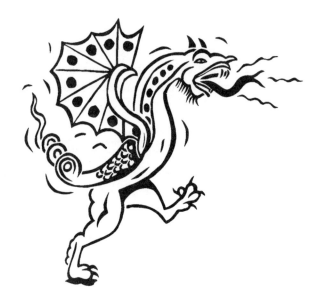

go through life quite happily on their own, reflecting their innate independence.

Compatibility: Dragons get on very well with most of the other animals—even with other Dragons. In fact, this unlikely pairing is one of the strongest, followed by Rats and Monkeys. Relationships with Horses and Sheep are likely to need plenty of work, and the least compatible animal is the Dog.

THE SNAKE

The Snake is in many ways a more subtle, and perhaps wiser, form of the Dragon. They are, to use a word so long associated with the famous Charlie Chan, 'inscrutable'. Snakes have an innate wisdom that seems to guide them away from trouble, which is just as well, because they absolutely adore the good life! Snakes like good food, good music, good everything: indeed, they'll even forgo a certain amount of comfort to savour top quality. Apart from gambling, which snakes should avoid, fortune favours the Snake, and he or she is likely to be very successful. In a partner, the Snake also looks for only the best. Once that partner has been found, they will not be easily parted.

Compatibility: Snakes are most compatible with Roosters, Oxen and other Snakes, but they are so subtle in their ways that they can form good relationships with those signs with which they have little in common, including Boars, Monkeys, Tigers and Horses.

THE HORSE

The wild mountain horse is all spirit and adventure, an animal that loves to run free and will defy attempts to tame it. This is the typical Horse person! Although they can be changeable or temperamental, Horses are generally cheerful creatures who gallop through life in a blur of fun and games. And despite being quite selfish and unpredictable, Horses have a unique ability to be popular and to succeed without any apparent preparation. The Horse's high spirits carry over into its love life, and Fire Horses in particular are considered more passionate than any other sign.

Compatibility: The Horse is compatible with just about anybody for a short time, and will probably fall in and out of love frequently. But when it comes to long-term relationships, his or her changeability can create a great deal of strain and take the gloss off any affair. Dogs, Tigers and Sheep make the best partners, while Rats, Snakes and Rabbits are unlikely to make lasting partners.

THE SHEEP

This is the gentlest of all the animals, good and kind and full of consideration for others. In fact, this makes Sheep fair game for more unscrupulous people, and their reticence to stand up and fight for their own rights leaves them vulnerable. But beware, when they do decide to fight, Sheep are a formidable foe! They can tend to be gloomy, but they're also very artistic, and often lucky. In relationships, they do best with someone who will provide the assertiveness they lack.

Compatibility: The Horse makes a great partner for the Sheep, with the Boar and Rabbit not far behind. Partnerships with other Sheep can be successful, but relationships with Rats, Tigers, Monkeys and Roosters are difficult and one with an Ox could result in disaster.

THE MONKEY

The Monkey is a charming character, clever and resourceful and not above distorting the facts to achieve his or her goal. Even if you get caught up in one of Monkey's deceptions (which was probably only devised to help you, anyway) you probably won't be able to stay angry for long. This charmer and indomitable trickster will soon have you and everybody else wrapped around his or her finger again. Don't try to keep up with the Monkey, its mental agility will leave most people floundering: just enjoy what you don't understand! It's sometimes difficult for Monkeys to direct special attention to just one person, which can make their love-life frustrating for both parties.

Compatibility: Monkeys love other Monkeys and delight in this mutual admiration. They usually form excellent relationships with Rats. Rarely do Tigers and Monkeys enjoy anything other an argument together.

THE ROOSTER

The Rooster is good with money and a good organiser, and is therefore inclined to strut its stuff and take charge of those around. This would be fine, except the Rooster will insist on letting everyone know just who is the boss, and with a curious blend of charm, wit and quite tactless critical observations will take centre stage at every opportunity. Indeed, there's a strong theatrical element to the Rooster which makes it difficult for others to find the real person beneath. The Rooster never does things in half-measures, and is either extremely happy or totally distressed. In the Rooster's love-life, it's all or nothing, love or hate.

Compatibility: The erratic nature of the Rooster makes for difficult relationships, with the Snake and the Ox the most likely candidates for lasting friendships. Other combinations can be difficult, particularly those with Dogs, Monkeys or other Roosters, and the Rabbit/Rooster pairing is a prime candidate for failure.

THE DOG

The Dog is the most fair-minded of the animal symbols, and seeks justice and fairness, not only for itself but for all those around it, defending its friends and righting wrongs with selfless energy. Just like the animal, the Dog person is the best friend one could possibly have. On the negative side, for all its intelligence, the Dog tends to see things in black and white, and is deeply suspicious of those who it does not know or whose motives seem unclear. In matters of the heart, Dogs are uncertain of new acquaintances, and will only form relationships slowly. Once formed, however, they are seldom broken.

Compatibility: When the initial reticence to become involved is overcome, Dogs get on reasonably well with most animals, and have a particularly good likelihood of success with Tigers and Horses. Problems could occur with Roosters, while Dragons present real difficulties. For younger Dogs, a relationship with a mature Rat can be the way to happiness.

THE BOAR

Under the rather rough exterior of the Boar is a decent person who enjoys the good things in life. He or she is fundamentally honest, loyal, and quite soft-hearted, characteristics which make Boars excellent friends. Boars like to have a good time, and don't bother to hide it! Tact is not the Boar's strong point, however, and he or she is unlikely to succeed where diplomacy is needed, although their other features generally bring success in their careers. The Boar is also generous, but expects friends to reciprocate: failure to do so will lead to a rapid cooling in the friendship or romance. Male and female Boars have strong sexual desires and enjoy physical relationships.

Compatibility: Rabbits and Sheep make good partners for Boars, as they are happy to provide the understanding in the relationship, while the Boar provides the passion. Other signs are generally reasonable, but Monkeys and other Boars make less likely partners while Snakes and Boars simply don't communicate at all.

Take some time to just share a kiss. Start with soft, gentle kisses on the lips and face and gradually allow yourself the pleasure of longer, more passionate kisses.

Go for a romantic walk holding hands.

I

Do you enjoy making love with your eyes opened or closed?

II

Describe a perfect head massage.

III

Do you need to have an orgasm in each love making session?

© 1989

Picnic Passion

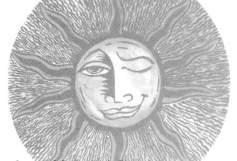

Is a picnic a form of foreplay? Certainly.

Imagine a secluded, leafy spot beside a waterfall. Perhaps you'd prefer an isolated beach or the splendour of a park. Enjoying the outdoors and simply being in the fresh air is an aphrodisiac: add food, wine, a tantalising companion and a relaxed frame of mind and your picnic will be a truly exhilarating experience.

Choose a picnic spot not too far away. Take some breezy music to play in the car as you make your way there. The food and wine are important. Light, easy-to-handle food with a touch of sophistication works best. Go for sexy food that you can hold in one hand and feed to your lover. Biscuits and cheese or pâté, chicken wings, fruit, chocolate—all of these are easy to prepare and fun to eat. Very heavy wines are out. And don't forget to take some mineral water as well, since picnics combined with bush or beach walks are often thirsty occasions.

Remember that picnics aren't just for kids. The picnic is

an important weapon in your seductive armoury, so why not start planning one now?

Between The Sheets 9
ABSURD SITUATIONS

Roll the die, and the highest score begins. Each number on the die represents an absurd sentence.

Each player rolls the die, reads out whatever number is thrown, and completes the telling of the absurd situation.

1) *Who would have thought that I'd be standing in the middle of Martin Place with my pants down around my ankles?*

2) *Stuck in a traffic jam on the freeway, my lover and I decided to break the monotony by having oral sex . . .*

3) *I was offered a million dollars for a one night stand and . . .*

4) *While making love in the toilet in a plane, we generated so much heat we set off an alarm . . .*

5) *I slipped outside my flat to get the paper, and the door slammed shut and locked. The only problem was that I didn't have a key and I was in my underwear . . .*

6) *After getting dumped by a wave at the beach I realised that my bathers had come off . . .*

Truth or dare

Answer these with your partner—if you dare . . .

How often would you like to perform oral sex?

A) More often

B) Less often

C) The same amount as now

D) Never

This probably won't come as a surprise . . . Nearly 50% of men would like oral sex more often. 59% of women are happy with 'the same amount as now'.

> Please darling, dear Ipsithilla,
>
> All my pleasure, my only attraction.
>
> Order me to you this afternoon
>
> And if you do order me, please arrange also
>
> That no one shall get in my way as I enter
>
> And don't you go off either at the last moment
>
> But stay at home and organise for us
>
> Nine copulations in a rapid series.
>
> If there's anything doing, send round immediately
>
> For here I am, lying on my bed;
>
> I have had my lunch, my thing sticks out of my tunic.
>
> CATULLUS (84–54 BC)

Teasers

Try your luck at guessing these cheeky picture puzzles. Answers are
written at the foot of the page.

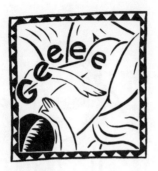

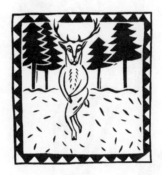

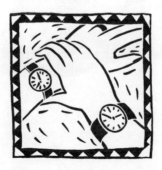

1. G-spot; 2. buck naked; 3. two-timing.

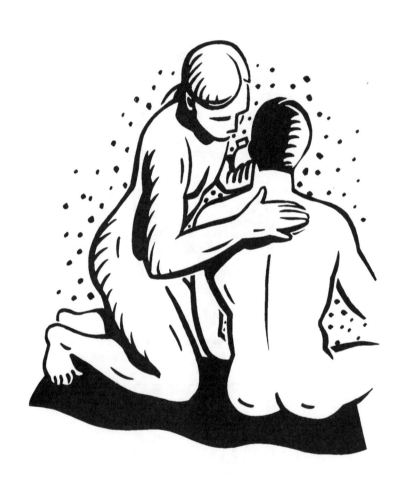

From Foreplay to Climax

Sex is great—the only thing that's better is more sex. And don't forget the old saying that there's no such thing as bad sex, only varying degrees of good sex. Trust, laughter and communication are the three basics to start off with. Keep them in mind and you'll get the best from each other in the sexual playground.

If you haven't already swapped the following secrets, here are some questions which will help you to understand each other's needs.

Describe what an orgasm feels like to you.

What is your greatest turn-on?

What is your favourite bit of foreplay?

Describe any fetishes you suspect, or know, you might have (dressing up? being turned on by shoes?).

What is the best sex you've both shared?

What is your most recent fantasy?

Describe what gives you the most pleasure during lovemaking.

Show where, and how, you like to be touched.

MAGIC MASSAGES

A massage is an intimate way to learn about your partner's sexuality. It's like taking a tour of their body: a learning experience for you, and fun for them! Try the following discovery trail, and, as you go, become attuned to your partner's sensual responses to see what works best.

HER

Begin by asking your partner to lie face-down naked on the bed. Warm your hands with baby oil, or a more exotic, scented oil if she prefers.

Start with the feet, rubbing the oil gently into the skin, alternating the strength of your fingers from very soft to firm again. Next, using your fingertips as sensuously as possible, work slowly up her calves to the back of the knees. At this point, you can switch to the back of the neck, spending some time here to ease and soothe away any aches and tension.

Now, work down over her shoulders and arms, digging your fingertips gently into the muscles. Pay the hands special attention. Then you can move to the rest of her body, starting on her shoulder blades. Ask your partner to turn over, and beginning on the lowest ribs, gently smooth your hands over them, out from the centre of the body to the side. Move slowly to the breasts, making the most of the sensitive nipples. Then work back downwards over her belly to the inner thighs. By this stage you should know how much she has enjoyed the massage!

HIM

Remember that men love a topless masseuse—or better still, a completely naked one! You can also try wearing something silky, which will feel gorgeous when it rubs against bare skin.

Begin by getting your partner to lie naked and face-down on the bed. Moisten your hands with a little baby oil to help the palms and fingertips slide smoothly over the skin.

Start by kneading his shoulders and upper back, where men store a lot of tension. Work hard on the places where he is experiencing muscle soreness, and that will help ease any pain and relax him.

Work slowly down his spine, prodding gently in between the bones. When you reach the base of the spine, use your outspread hands to stroke his buttocks lovingly.

Now, work up and down the insides of his thighs, and the back of his calves. Only after this should you let him turn over . . . You'll probably find he is eager for much more

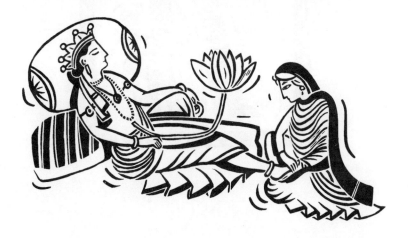

than foreplay by now, but you can prolong the fun a little longer by stroking his nipples and massaging the muscles of his belly.

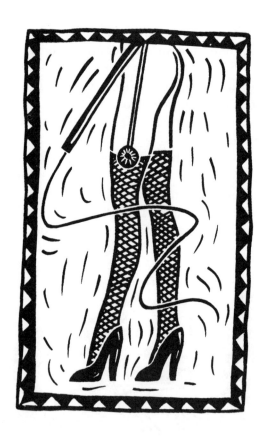

Romance

Ideally, romance should be coupled with physical love so that a love affair retains that special magic. Unfortunately, romantic gestures are usually the first casualties of the long-term relationship. Try discussing these questions together:

What is the most romantic thing your lover has done for you?

Would you send your lover some flowers tomorrow?

What would you write in a love letter?

Would you consider starting your relationship over again by dating your lover?

What are the five most wonderful things you feel about your lover?

Would you now be embarrassed to do the squishy things you did at the beginning of your relationship?

Would you enjoy a candle-lit dinner for two?

Would you enjoy a dirty weekend together?

Solutions to Crosswords and Quizzes

LOVERS' CROSSWORD SOLUTION

Crossword solution grid:

¹C	A	N	E	D		³V	⁴A	⁵N	⁶I	T	Y		⁷M	
A			²D	A		⁸E	R	O	S			⁹T	⁹A	¹⁰B
¹¹R	¹²O	¹³M	A	N	¹⁴T	I	C			¹⁵F	A	I	R	Y
¹⁶E	R	A		¹⁷C	A	N		¹⁸C	¹⁹U	P	I	D	E	
²⁰S	E	²¹N	S	E	S		O		²²A	R	²³O	M	A	
S		²⁴E	S	S	E	²⁵N	C	E	S		²⁶R	O	S	E
	²⁷F	U	N		E		²⁸O	K		²⁹S	³⁰C	E	N	T
³¹L	A		³²S	A	L	T		³³I	R		³⁴A	S	K	³⁵K
N		U			³⁶T	A	B	O	O					I
³⁷T	O	A	³⁸S	T	S		I		³⁹N	O	V	E	L	⁴⁰S
⁴¹L	A		A		⁴²C	L	E	A	N				⁴³I	S
⁴⁴A	S	P		⁴⁵E	V	I	L		⁴⁶T	E	M	⁴⁷P	T	
⁴⁸B	Y		⁴⁹B	E		⁵⁰O	⁵¹T	H	E	R		⁵²A	T	M
I		⁵³E	⁵⁴R	R		⁵⁵T	A	L		⁵⁶A	T	E		
⁵⁷A	I	M	⁵⁸A	N	C	H	O	V	Y		⁵⁹M	E	R	E

LOVERS' LITTLE CROSSWORD SOLUTION

1	2	3	4	5	6	7	8	9	10	11	12
M	A	N	G	O	█	C	A	P	O	T	E
█	G	O	O	D	█	G	A	P	█	█	R
T	E	D	D	Y	█	B	O	L	E	R	O
A	S	█	I	L	Y	A	█	█	N	I	T
N	█	█	V	█	Z	O	O	█	█	P	I
G	O	█	A	F	F	A	I	R	█	E	C
O	W	L	█	O	R	A	L	█	█	N	█
█	N	E	A	R	E	R	█	A	M	█	P
█	█	T	E	N	█	A	M	O	U	R	█
F	O	B	█	I	C	A	R	U	S	█	A
E	N	O	U	G	H	█	E	S	S	A	Y
Z	E	N	█	N	█	U	S	E	█	█	S

HOW DO YOU RATE AS A LOVER?

SCORING

1)	a4 b3 c2 d1
2)	a3 b1 c4 d2
3)	a1 b2 c3 d4
4)	a2 b1 c4 d3
5)	a2 b1 c3 d4
6)	a1 b3 c4 d2
7)	a2 b3 c4 d1
8)	a3 b4 c2 d1
9)	a2 b4 c1 d3
10)	a3 b1 c4 d2
11)	a2 b4 c3 d1
12)	a2 b4 c1 d3
13)	a4 b2 c3 d1
14)	a1 b2 c3 d4
15)	a2 b1 c3 d4
16)	a3 b4 c2 d1
17)	a3 b1 c4 d2
18)	a3 b4 c2 d1
19)	a3 b1 c4 d2
20)	a2 b4 c3 d1

60–80

We don't need to worry about you, do we? You're not scared to be spontaneous, adventurous and downright sexy! You care about your partner but you know what you like, too.

40–60

No problem here! You are a thoughtful and fairly relaxed lover. Just loosen up a bit more and remember to listen to your partner.

30–40

Don't be so tense! It takes two to tango! Rent some naughty vids and let it all hang out!

1–30

Dear oh dear oh dear! Your heart—and other parts—are just not in this, are they? Get out of that thermal underwear, stop counting sheep and get into it! Why not try some good sex manuals, or, better still, buy the Foreplay board game!

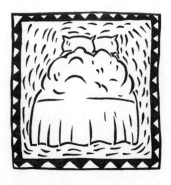

Scoring

1)	a4 b3 c2 d1
2)	a1 b2 c4 d3
3)	a3 b4 c2 d1
4)	a4 b3 c2 d1
5)	a1 b3 c4 d2
6)	a4 b2 c1 d3
7)	a2 b4 c1 d3
8)	a4 b3 c2 d1
9)	a1 b4 c2 d3
10)	a1 b4 c3 d2
11)	a1 b4 c3 d2
12)	a1 b4 c2 d3
13)	a3 b2 c4 d1
14)	a1 b4 c3 d2
15)	a3 b4 c2 d1
16)	a4 b1 c3 d2
17)	a2 b3 c4 d1
18)	a3 b2 c1 d4
19)	a4 b1 c2 d3
20)	a3 b2 c1 d4

60–80

Wow! Aren't you lucky! Your partner is a lover of Olympian proportions: sexy, giving, makes you feel great—just make sure you give as good as you get.

40–60

Romance and sex go hand in hand with your lover. Keep that spark going and this relationship will stay simmering.

20–40

OK, so sexually your partner might be a few condoms short of the box. Be more encouraging, take the initiative yourself. Together you can lift the lustful limits on your love life.

0–20

What are you doing with this person? A stone statue would be more erotic, and certainly a lot warmer. Get out of it and find a new bedmate! There are plenty of others out there waiting to take you on the magic carpet ride.

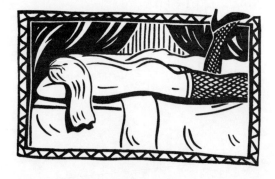

How Confident Are You Sexually?

Scoring

1)	a1 b3 c4 d2
2)	a2 b3 c1 d4
3)	a2 b1 c4 d3
4)	a4 b1 c3 d2
5)	a1 b4 c3 d2
6)	a2 b3 c4 d1
7)	a4 b2 c1 d3
8)	a4 b3 c2 d1
9)	a2 b4 c1 d3
10)	a1 b3 c2 d4
11)	a4 b1 c2 d3
12)	a1 b3 c2 d4
13)	a4 b1 c2 d3
14)	a2 b3 c4 d1
15)	a4 b2 c3 d1
16)	a3 b1 c4 d2
17)	a2 b4 c1 d3
18)	a3 b4 c2 d1
19)	a1 b2 c3 d4
20)	a2 b1 c4 d3

60–80

You don't know what the word shy means! You are self-confident and know what you want, not only from yourself but also from your partner. Although finding a lover to match your confidence could be a problem. Good luck!

40–60

You're doing well! You are happy with your sex life, and fairly confident about your sexuality. Just relax, keep up those 'confidence' vibes and understand that sex is not just bed and intercourse.

20–30

Get to know your own body better, and build up your sexual confidence by doing some trust exercises with your partner. As the trust in your relationship deepens, so will the belief in your self. Talk more with your partner about different aspects of romance and sex.

1–20

You'll have to build up your self esteem in your everyday life before trying to conquer your sexual confidence. Recognise the good points about you, know that other people like you. Praise the positive things you do and learn to like yourself. Make sure you choose confidence-boosting lovers, not confidence-destroying ones.